DR. RICHARD CALDWELL

The Heart-Healthy Cookbook For Seniors 2024

Tasty Low-fat and Low-Sodium Recipes to Reduce Blood Pressure and Cholesterol for Improving Heart Health and Improve Overall Wellbeing. Includes a 30-Day Meal Plan

First edition

This book was professionally typeset on Reedsy.
Find out more at reedsy.com

"You have only one heart, so make sure that you give all your attention to its well-being."

Contents

Chapter 1: Introduction   1

    1.1 Why Heart Health Matters for Seniors   1

    1.2 The Importance of a Heart-Healthy Diet   2

Chapter 2: Understanding Heart-Healthy Ingredients   4

    2.1 Incorporating Whole Grains   4

    2.2 Choosing Lean Proteins   6

    2.3 Embracing Heart-Friendly Fats   7

    2.4 Power of Fresh Fruits and Vegetables   9

Chapter 3: Essential Cooking Techniques   12

    3.1 Heart-Friendly Cooking Oils   12

    3.2 Flavoring Without Excess Sodium   14

    3.3 Smart Substitutions for Healthier Meals   16

    3.4 Portion Control for Seniors   18

Chapter 4: Breakfasts to Start Your Day Right   21

    Classic Overnight Oats   21

    Spinach and Feta Egg Muffins   22

    Quinoa Breakfast Bowl   23

    Smashed Avocado on Whole-Grain Toast with Cherry Tomatoes   24

    Blueberry and Almond Butter Smoothie   24

    Sweet Potato Hash with Eggs   25

    Banana Walnut Pancakes   26

    Apple Cinnamon Chia Pudding   27

    Veggie and Hummus Breakfast Wrap   28

    Pomegranate and Pistachio Yogurt Parfait   29

    Salmon and Avocado Bagel   29

    Coconut and Mango Chia Seed Smoothie Bowl   30

Tomato Basil Mozzarella Frittata 31
Almond Butter Banana Toast 32
Mediterranean Breakfast Bowl 32
Chapter 5: Nourishing Lunches 34
Grilled Chicken Salad with Mixed Greens 34
Quinoa and Black Bean Bowl 35
Mediterranean Chickpea Wrap 35
Salmon and Quinoa Stuffed Bell Peppers 36
Vegetarian Buddha Bowl 37
Caprese Avocado Toast 38
Turkey and Veggie Lettuce Wraps 38
Whole Wheat Veggie Pasta Salad 39
Sweet Potato and Black Bean Quesadilla 40
Greek Quinoa Salad with Grilled Shrimp 41
Chickpea and Vegetable Stir-Fry 42
Roasted Vegetable and Hummus Wrap 42
Tuna and White Bean Salad 43
Cauliflower Rice Bowl with Teriyaki Tofu 44
Pesto Chicken Quinoa Bowl 45
Chapter 6: Wholesome Dinners 46
Baked Lemon Herb Chicken with Roasted Vegetables 46
Lentil and Vegetable Curry with Brown Rice 47
Grilled Salmon with Quinoa and Asparagus 48
Spinach and Feta Stuffed Chicken Breast with Sweet
Potato Mash 49
Chickpea and Spinach Stew over Couscous 49
Teriyaki Tofu Stir-Fry with Broccoli and Brown Rice 50
Mediterranean Baked Cod with Tomato and Olive Relish 51
Quinoa and Black Bean Stuffed Peppers 52
Shrimp and Avocado Salad with Citrus Vinaigrette 53
Butternut Squash and Kale Risotto 54
Turkey and Vegetable Skewers with Quinoa Pilaf 55
Eggplant Parmesan with Whole Wheat Spaghetti 56

Balsamic Glazed Chicken Thighs with Brussels Sprouts   57
Zucchini Noodles with Pesto and Cherry Tomatoes   57
Beef and Vegetable Stir-Fry with Cauliflower Rice   58
Chapter 7: Sides and Snacks   60
Roasted Garlic Hummus with Veggie Sticks   60
Baked Sweet Potato Fries   61
Caprese Skewers   61
Guacamole with Whole Grain Tortilla Chips   62
Cucumber and Greek Yogurt Dip   63
Quinoa-Stuffed Mushrooms   63
Cheese and Whole Wheat Crackers Platter   64
Roasted Chickpeas   65
Greek Salad Skewers   65
Veggie Spring Rolls with Peanut Dipping Sauce   66
Baked Parmesan Zucchini Chips   67
Mixed Berry Yogurt Parfait   68
Salsa and Black Bean Corn Cups   68
Spicy Edamame   69
Baba Ganoush with Pita Bread   70
Chapter 8: Desserts with a Heart-Healthy Twist   71
Dark Chocolate-Dipped Strawberries   71
Oatmeal Banana Cookies   72
Greek Yogurt and Berry Popsicles   72
Avocado Chocolate Mousse   73
Almond Flour Blueberry Muffins   74
Dark Chocolate-Dipped Strawberries   74
Oatmeal Banana Cookies   75
Greek Yogurt and Berry Popsicles   76
Avocado Chocolate Mousse   76
Almond Flour Blueberry Muffins   77
Mango Sorbet   78
Pecan and Date Energy Bites   79
Chapter 9: Beverages for Heart Health   80

Green Tea Infusion with Citrus Twist ... 80

Berry Blast Smoothie with Flaxseed ... 81

Hibiscus and Ginger Iced Tea ... 81

Kale and Pineapple Detox Juice ... 82

Golden Turmeric Latte ... 83

Watermelon Mint Refresher ... 84

Blueberry and Almond Milk Protein Shake ... 84

Cucumber Basil Sparkling Water ... 85

Cranberry and Orange Zest Mocktail ... 86

Matcha Green Tea Smoothie ... 86

Beetroot and Berry Power Juice ... 87

Chia Seed Lemonade with Honey ... 88

Chapter 10: Meal Planning and Grocery Shopping Tips ... 89

10.1 Building a Heart-Healthy Grocery List ... 89

10.2 Weekly Meal Planning for Seniors ... 92

10.3 30-Day Heart-Healthy Meal Plan for Seniors ... 94

Week 1: ... 94

Week 2: ... 98

Week 3: ... 101

Week 4: ... 104

Chapter 11: Maintaining a Heart-Healthy Lifestyle ... 109

11.1 Incorporating Physical Activity ... 109

11.2 Stress Management and Its Impact on Heart Health ... 111

11.3 Regular Health Checkups for Seniors ... 113

Chapter 12: Conclusion ... 118

12.1 Celebrating a Heart-Healthy Lifestyle ... 118

12.2 Final Note ... 120

Chapter 1: Introduction

My name is Dr. Richard Caldwell, a seasoned professional with over 15 years of dedicated experience in the field of cardiology. Throughout my career, I have been driven by a profound commitment to improving the cardiovascular health of individuals, particularly seniors. This cookbook represents not only my expertise in cardiology but also my passion for creating a resource that empowers you to embrace a heart-healthy lifestyle through the joy of cooking. Drawing upon a wealth of clinical experiences, I aim to convey the increasing importance of adopting proactive measures to promote cardiovascular well-being. Through these pages, I hope to inspire a deeper understanding of how prioritizing heart health can positively influence the overall quality of life for our beloved seniors.

1.1 Why Heart Health Matters for Seniors

In the graceful dance of aging, the heartbeat becomes not just a rhythm of life but a poignant melody that underscores the symphony of well-being. Understanding why heart health is paramount for seniors requires a nuanced exploration of the physiological intricacies that accompany the passage of time.

As we gracefully grow older, the cardiovascular system undergoes changes that demand our attention. Arteries may lose some elasticity, blood vessels might become less pliant, and the heart itself may experience alterations in structure and function. These subtle shifts, while part of the natural aging process, underscore the necessity of adopting a proactive stance towards heart health.

A healthy heart is not merely a pumping organ; it is the conductor of vitality, orchestrating the flow of life-giving oxygen and nutrients to every nook and cranny of the body. Maintaining cardiovascular health in the senior years is pivotal for sustaining energy levels, cognitive function, and overall physical well-being.

Furthermore, the heart is a sentinel against the encroachment of cardiovascular diseases, which become more prevalent with age. Conditions such as hypertension, atherosclerosis, and heart failure may manifest, necessitating a deliberate and informed approach to lifestyle choices.

1.2 The Importance of a Heart-Healthy Diet

As a seasoned cardiologist, my years of professional engagement underscore the pivotal connection between dietary choices and cardiovascular well-being. A heart-healthy diet is not a mere culinary preference; it is a strategic investment in sustained health, longevity, and the prevention of cardiovascular diseases that may become more prevalent in the senior years.

Let us embark on a journey to dissect the elements of a heart-healthy diet, understanding that it goes beyond a mere reduction in saturated fats or sodium. At its core, a heart-healthy diet is a harmonious ensemble of nutrient-dense foods that support the intricate machinery of the cardiovascular system.

Key Components of a Heart-Healthy Diet:

Incorporating Whole Grains: Whole grains such as quinoa, brown rice, and oats bring not only a delightful variety of textures and flavors but also a rich supply of fiber, vitamins, and minerals crucial for heart health.

Choosing Lean Proteins: The protein choices we make play a crucial role in cardiovascular health. Opting for lean proteins like fish, poultry, legumes, and tofu ensures a balance between essential amino acids and heart-friendly fats.

Embracing Heart-Friendly Fats: Not all fats are created equal, and embracing the right kind is paramount. Incorporating sources of omega-3 fatty acids, such as fatty fish, flaxseeds, and walnuts, contributes to a heart-healthy lipid profile.

Power of Fresh Fruits and Vegetables: Colorful and nutrient-packed fruits and vegetables are not just culinary adornments; they are the cornerstone of a heart-healthy diet, providing antioxidants, vitamins, and minerals that fortify cardiovascular resilience.

Chapter 2: Understanding Heart-Healthy Ingredients

In this chapter, we embark on an in-depth exploration of the fundamental elements that constitute a heart-healthy diet. As we delve into this multifaceted journey, we aim to unravel the intricacies of ingredient choices, providing you with comprehensive insights and practical strategies that seamlessly integrate into your culinary repertoire, promoting not just flavor but enduring cardiovascular well-being.

2.1 Incorporating Whole Grains

Whole grains are the unsung heroes of a heart-healthy diet, offering a wealth of nutritional benefits that extend far beyond mere sustenance. In this section, we will delve into the significance of incorporating whole grains into your meals, understanding their unique qualities, and discovering practical ways to make them a delicious and integral part of your daily diet.

The Nutritional Powerhouse of Whole Grains:

Whole grains encompass a variety of grains that have retained their entire kernel, including the bran, germ, and endosperm. This preservation of the whole grain structure results in a nutritional powerhouse, rich in fiber, vitamins, minerals, and antioxidants. The benefits of whole grains extend to stabilizing blood sugar levels, promoting digestive health, and contributing to weight management—crucial aspects of cardiovascular well-being.

Exploring Different Whole Grains:

Dive into the diverse world of whole grains, each bringing its unique flavor, texture, and nutritional profile to the table. From the earthy notes of quinoa to the nutty richness of brown rice and the hearty goodness of oats, we will explore a variety of options. Discovering the versatility of whole grains allows you to tailor your choices to suit different dishes, making them a delightful addition to your culinary repertoire.

Practical Tips for Incorporation:

Incorporating whole grains into your meals doesn't have to be a complex endeavor. This section provides practical tips and creative ideas to seamlessly integrate whole grains into your diet. Whether it's substituting refined grains with whole grains in your favorite recipes or exploring new dishes that highlight the unique characteristics of different grains, you'll find accessible ways to make whole grains a staple in your kitchen.

Building Balanced Meals:

Understanding how to build balanced meals with whole grains as a foundation is key to deriving maximum benefits. We'll discuss portion control, pairing whole grains with lean proteins and an array of colorful vegetables, and creating meals that not only satisfy your taste buds but also contribute to overall heart health.

As we navigate the world of whole grains, the goal is to empower you with the knowledge and inspiration to make informed choices. Whether you're a seasoned cook or just starting on your culinary journey, incorporating whole grains into your diet is a small yet impactful step towards fostering a heart-healthy lifestyle. Join me in embracing the nutritional richness and culinary versatility that whole grains bring to the table.

2.2 Choosing Lean Proteins

The type of proteins we choose plays a crucial role in shaping the cardiovascular impact of our diet. This section is dedicated to unraveling the nuances of lean proteins—options that offer the essential building blocks for our body without the excess baggage of unhealthy fats.

Understanding Lean Proteins:

Lean proteins are characterized by their relatively low-fat content compared to other protein sources. They provide a concentrated source of essential amino acids, vital for muscle maintenance, immune function, and overall well-being. Incorporating lean proteins into your diet supports cardiovascular health by helping to manage cholesterol levels and maintain a healthy weight.

Exploring Lean Protein Options:

This section takes a closer look at a variety of lean protein sources, each bringing its unique nutritional benefits and culinary versatility. From the omega-3 fatty acids-rich goodness of fish like salmon and trout to the lean protein punch of poultry, and plant-powered alternatives like legumes and tofu, we'll explore options suitable for various dietary preferences.

Practical Integration into Meals:

Incorporating lean proteins into your meals need not be a daunting task. Practical tips and simple cooking techniques will be discussed to make the integration seamless and enjoyable. Whether you're grilling, baking, or sautéing, understanding how to prepare lean proteins ensures that your meals are not only heart-healthy but also satisfying to the palate.

Balancing Protein Intake:

Understanding the importance of balanced nutrition, this section will guide you in incorporating lean proteins into a well-rounded meal. We'll discuss portion control, pairing proteins with complementary grains and vegetables, and creating meals that provide sustained energy while supporting heart health.

Making Informed Choices:

As we navigate the landscape of lean proteins, the goal is to empower you with the knowledge to make informed choices that align with your dietary preferences and health goals. Whether you're looking to diversify your protein sources or simply exploring new ways to prepare your favorite lean meats, this section is a practical guide to incorporating heart-healthy proteins into your everyday meals.

Join me in exploring the world of lean proteins—a journey that goes beyond nutritional benefits, encompassing the delight of diverse flavors and the satisfaction of contributing to your overall cardiovascular well-being. Let's make conscious choices in selecting proteins that nourish not only our bodies but also our hearts.

2.3 Embracing Heart-Friendly Fats

Contrary to the notion that all fats are detrimental, this section is dedicated to unraveling the concept of heart-friendly fats—essential components of a balanced diet that contribute to cardiovascular well-being.

Understanding Heart-Friendly Fats:

Heart-friendly fats, also known as unsaturated fats, play a pivotal role in supporting heart health. Unlike saturated and trans fats, which are associated with adverse cardiovascular effects, heart-friendly fats come in two primary forms: monounsaturated fats and polyunsaturated fats. These fats have been linked to lower cholesterol levels and a reduced risk of heart disease when incorporated into a balanced diet.

Exploring Heart-Friendly Fat Sources:

This section delves into the rich sources of heart-friendly fats, guiding you through a diverse array of options. From the omega-3 fatty acids abundant in fatty fish like salmon and flaxseeds to the monounsaturated haven of avocados and olive oil, we'll explore the nutritional benefits and culinary versatility of incorporating these fats into your meals.

Cooking with Heart-Friendly Fats:

Practical tips on cooking with heart-friendly fats will be shared to make the integration seamless and enjoyable. Whether you're sautéing, drizzling, or using heart-friendly oils in your baking, understanding the various cooking applications ensures that you not only enhance the flavors of your dishes but also support your cardiovascular health.

Balancing Fat Intake:

While heart-friendly fats offer numerous benefits, balance is key. This section provides insights into maintaining a balanced fat intake within the context of an overall healthy diet. Understanding portion control and incorporating a variety of heart-friendly fat sources into your meals contributes to both flavor diversity and heart health.

Incorporating Heart-Friendly Fats into Meals:

We'll discuss practical ways to incorporate heart-friendly fats into your everyday meals, ensuring that the transition to a heart-conscious diet is not only manageable but also enjoyable. From salad dressings to cooking oils, discover how small adjustments in your kitchen can lead to significant benefits for your heart.

As we embark on this journey of embracing heart-friendly fats, the goal is to demystify their role in our diet and empower you with the knowledge to make conscious and enjoyable choices. Join me in discovering the richness of flavors and the nutritional benefits that heart-friendly fats bring to the table, making every meal a delightful and heart-conscious experience.

2.4 Power of Fresh Fruits and Vegetables

In our exploration of heart-healthy ingredients, we now turn our attention to the vibrant and nutrient-packed world of fresh fruits and vegetables. This section is dedicated to unraveling the numerous benefits that these colorful gems offer, not just for the palate but for overall cardiovascular well-being.

Nutritional Bounty of Fresh Produce:

Fresh fruits and vegetables are nature's nutritional powerhouses, offering an array of vitamins, minerals, fiber, and antioxidants. Their consumption has been linked to a reduced risk of heart disease, lower blood pressure, and improved overall health. Understanding the nutritional bounty that fresh produce provides is essential for cultivating a heart-healthy diet.

Diverse Range of Fresh Produce:

This section delves into the diverse world of fresh fruits and vegetables, celebrating the spectrum of flavors, textures, and nutritional profiles they bring to our plates. From the crispness of leafy greens to the sweetness of berries and the versatility of various vegetables, we'll explore how incorporating a variety of fresh produce can add vibrancy to your meals while supporting your heart health.

Benefits Beyond Nutrition:

Beyond their nutritional content, fresh fruits and vegetables offer additional health benefits. Their high water content contributes to hydration, while their fiber content aids in digestion and weight management—both crucial elements for cardiovascular health. This section highlights the holistic advantages of embracing fresh produce as an integral part of your daily diet.

Practical Tips for Incorporation:

Practical tips for easily incorporating fresh fruits and vegetables into your meals will be shared. Whether you're looking to boost your daily intake through snacks, salads, or complementary sides to your main dishes, this section provides practical strategies to make fresh produce a seamless and enjoyable part of your culinary routine.

Colorful Plate for a Healthy Heart:

Creating a colorful plate by including a variety of fruits and vegetables is not just visually appealing but also a practical approach to ensuring a broad spectrum of nutrients. We'll discuss how to balance different colors and types of produce to create meals that are not only nutritious but also delightful to the senses.

As we navigate the vast array of fresh fruits and vegetables, the goal is to inspire you to view them not just as ingredients but as essential contributors to your heart health. Join me in embracing the vibrant and wholesome world of fresh produce, making every meal a celebration of flavors, nutrition, and a healthier heart.

Chapter 3: Essential Cooking Techniques

As we continue our culinary journey toward heart-healthy living, Chapter 3 serves as a practical guide, focusing on essential cooking techniques that empower you to create flavorful and nutritious meals. Whether you're a seasoned chef or just beginning your cooking adventure, mastering these techniques lays the foundation for a diverse and heart-conscious kitchen.

3.1 Heart-Friendly Cooking Oils

The choice of cooking oils plays a pivotal role in determining the overall nutritional profile of your dishes. This section dives into the world of heart-friendly cooking oils, shedding light on the diverse options that not only enhance flavors but also contribute to cardiovascular well-being.

Understanding Heart-Friendly Cooking Oils:

Heart-friendly cooking oils are those that are rich in unsaturated fats, particularly monounsaturated and polyunsaturated fats, and low in saturated and trans fats. These oils have been associated with promoting heart health by helping to lower bad cholesterol (LDL) levels and supporting overall cardiovascular well-being.

Key Heart-Friendly Oils:

Olive Oil: Extra virgin olive oil, with its robust flavor and antioxidant properties, is a staple in heart-healthy cooking. It contains monounsaturated fats and has been linked to various cardiovascular benefits.

Avocado Oil: Extracted from avocados, this oil is rich in monounsaturated fats and boasts a high smoke point, making it suitable for sautéing and roasting.

Canola Oil: With a mild flavor and a high smoke point, canola oil is a versatile option for a range of cooking techniques. It is low in saturated fat and a good source of omega-3 fatty acids.

Grapeseed Oil: Known for its neutral taste and high smoke point, grapeseed oil is rich in polyunsaturated fats, contributing to heart health.

Flaxseed Oil: A source of omega-3 fatty acids, flaxseed oil is best used in dressings and sauces due to its low smoke point.

Choosing the Right Oil for the Right Dish:

Understanding the smoke points and flavor profiles of different heart-friendly oils is crucial. Olive oil, for instance, is excellent for drizzling over salads or dipping bread, while avocado oil's high smoke point makes it ideal for high-heat cooking methods like sautéing and roasting.

Practical Tips for Usage:

This section provides practical tips for incorporating heart-friendly oils into your cooking routine. Whether you're aiming to boost the flavor of a dish or seeking the health benefits associated with these oils, understanding how to use them effectively ensures a seamless integration into your heart-conscious kitchen.

Balancing Fat Intake:

While heart-friendly oils offer health benefits, moderation is key. This section emphasizes the importance of balancing fat intake, considering the overall composition of your diet. By making informed choices about cooking oils, you contribute to a balanced and heart-healthy culinary approach.

3.2 Flavoring Without Excess Sodium

The choice of cooking oils plays a pivotal role in determining the overall nutritional profile of your dishes. This section dives into the world of heart-friendly cooking oils, shedding light on the diverse options that not only enhance flavors but also contribute to cardiovascular well-being.

Understanding Heart-Friendly Cooking Oils:

Heart-friendly cooking oils are those that are rich in unsaturated fats, particularly monounsaturated and polyunsaturated fats, and low in saturated and trans fats. These oils have been associated with promoting heart health by helping to lower bad cholesterol (LDL) levels and supporting overall cardiovascular well-being.

Key Heart-Friendly Oils:

Olive Oil: Extra virgin olive oil, with its robust flavor and antioxidant properties, is a staple in heart-healthy cooking. It contains monounsaturated fats and has been linked to various cardiovascular benefits.

Avocado Oil: Extracted from avocados, this oil is rich in monounsaturated fats and boasts a high smoke point, making it suitable for sautéing and roasting.

Canola Oil: With a mild flavor and a high smoke point, canola oil is a versatile option for a range of cooking techniques. It is low in saturated fat and a good source of omega-3 fatty acids.

Grapeseed Oil: Known for its neutral taste and high smoke point, grapeseed oil is rich in polyunsaturated fats, contributing to heart health.

Flaxseed Oil: A source of omega-3 fatty acids, flaxseed oil is best used in dressings and sauces due to its low smoke point.

Choosing the Right Oil for the Right Dish:

Understanding the smoke points and flavor profiles of different heart-friendly oils is crucial. Olive oil, for instance, is excellent for drizzling over salads or dipping bread, while avocado oil's high smoke point makes it ideal for high-heat cooking methods like sautéing and roasting.

Practical Tips for Usage:

This section provides practical tips for incorporating heart-friendly oils into your cooking routine. Whether you're aiming to boost the flavor of a dish or seeking the health benefits associated with these oils, understanding how to use them effectively ensures a seamless integration into your heart-conscious kitchen.

Balancing Fat Intake:

While heart-friendly oils offer health benefits, moderation is key. This section emphasizes the importance of balancing fat intake, considering the overall composition of your diet. By making informed choices about cooking oils, you contribute to a balanced and heart-healthy culinary approach.

3.3 Smart Substitutions for Healthier Meals

In the pursuit of a heart-healthy kitchen, the ability to make smart substitutions is a culinary skill that can significantly impact the nutritional profile of your meals. This section is dedicated to exploring practical and delicious alternatives, allowing you to create healthier versions of your favorite dishes without compromising on flavor.

Understanding Smart Substitutions:

Smart substitutions involve replacing ingredients with healthier alternatives to reduce saturated fats, sodium, and overall calorie content. These substitutions aim to enhance the nutritional value of your meals, contributing to better heart health without sacrificing taste.

1. Whole Grains for Refined Grains:

Swap refined grains for whole grains to increase the fiber, vitamins, and minerals in your diet. Choose brown rice over white, whole wheat pasta instead of regular pasta, and opt for whole-grain bread to add nutritional depth to your meals.

2. Lean Proteins in Place of Fatty Cuts:

Choose lean protein sources to reduce saturated fats and calories. Opt for skinless poultry, lean cuts of meat, fish, legumes, and tofu. These alternatives provide essential amino acids without the excess unhealthy fats.

3. Heart-Friendly Oils Instead of Saturated Fats:

Replace saturated fats with heart-friendly oils like olive oil, canola oil, or avocado oil. These oils are rich in unsaturated fats and offer cardiovascular benefits while maintaining the integrity of your dishes.

4. Greek Yogurt for Sour Cream or Mayonnaise:

Greek yogurt is a versatile substitute for sour cream or mayonnaise in various recipes. It adds a creamy texture with less saturated fat and more protein. Use it in dips, dressings, or as a topping for a healthier twist.

5. Fresh Herbs and Spices Instead of Salt:

Reduce sodium intake by flavoring your dishes with fresh herbs and spices instead of salt. Herbs like basil, cilantro, and thyme, along with spices such as cumin and paprika, add depth and complexity without the need for excess salt.

6. Nutritional Sweeteners Instead of Refined Sugar:

Choose natural sweeteners like honey, maple syrup, or agave nectar to replace refined sugars. These alternatives add sweetness with additional nutrients, and their complex flavors can enhance the overall taste of your desserts and beverages.

7. Nut Butter in Place of Butter or Margarine:

Swap traditional butter or margarine with nut butter, such as almond or peanut butter. These alternatives provide healthy fats, protein, and a rich flavor profile without the saturated fats found in some traditional spreads.

8. Whole Fruit Instead of Fruit Juices:

Opt for whole fruits over fruit juices to increase fiber intake and reduce added sugars. Whole fruits retain their natural fiber, vitamins, and antioxidants, providing a more wholesome option for snacks or as part of your meals.

3.4 Portion Control for Seniors

As we tailor our approach to heart-healthy living, understanding the significance of portion control becomes paramount, especially for our senior community. This section is dedicated to exploring the principles of portion control, offering practical insights and strategies that align with the unique nutritional needs of seniors, and ensuring a balanced and heart-conscious dietary approach.

Importance of Portion Control for Seniors:

Portion control is a crucial aspect of maintaining a healthy lifestyle, particularly for seniors. As our bodies age, changes in metabolism and activity levels make it essential to pay closer attention to the quantity of food consumed. Proper portion control helps manage weight, control blood sugar levels, and reduce the risk of cardiovascular issues—all vital considerations for seniors.

Understanding Appropriate Portion Sizes:

This section guides recognizing appropriate portion sizes for different food groups. By understanding the right balance of proteins, carbohydrates, fats, and vegetables, seniors can make informed choices that support overall well-being.

1. Protein-Rich Foods:
   Aim for a portion of lean protein, such as fish, poultry, beans, or tofu, equivalent to the size of a palm.
   Prioritize variety to ensure a range of essential amino acids.

2. Whole Grains:
   Choose whole grains like brown rice or quinoa and portion them to fit within a cupped hand.
   Whole grains contribute to stable blood sugar levels and satiety.

3. Healthy Fats:
   Incorporate heart-friendly fats, like olive oil or avocados, in moderation. Limit portions to about a thumb-sized serving.
   These fats provide flavor and nutritional benefits without excess calories.

4. Vegetables:
   Load up on vegetables, aiming for half of your plate to be filled with colorful and nutrient-dense options.
   Vegetables are rich in vitamins, minerals, and fiber.

5. Fruits:
   Choose whole fruits and keep portions in check to manage sugar intake.
   Berries, apples, and citrus fruits are excellent choices for heart health.

Practical Tips for Portion Control:

This section offers practical tips tailored to the senior demographic, considering factors such as appetite changes, dietary restrictions, and nutritional needs. Strategies include:

- Using smaller plates to create visual cues for appropriate portions.
- Listening to hunger and fullness cues to avoid overeating.
- Engaging in mindful eating practices to savor each bite and recognize satisfaction.

Adapting to Lifestyle Changes:

Lifestyle changes, such as decreased activity levels or alterations in appetite, are common among seniors. This section provides insights into adapting portion control strategies to accommodate these changes, ensuring that nutritional needs are met while maintaining a healthy balance.

By embracing the principles of portion control tailored to the needs of seniors, we aim to foster a heart-healthy approach that is both sustainable and enjoyable. Join me in navigating the nuanced landscape of portion control, empowering seniors to make informed choices that contribute to their overall well-being and heart health.

Chapter 4: Breakfasts to Start Your Day Right

Classic Overnight Oats

Ingredients:

- 1/2 cup rolled oats
- 1/2 cup milk (dairy or plant-based)
- 1/2 cup Greek yogurt
- 1 tablespoon chia seeds
- 1 tablespoon honey or maple syrup
- 1/2 teaspoon vanilla extract
- Pinch of salt

Instructions:

1. In a jar or container, combine rolled oats, milk, Greek yogurt, chia seeds, honey or maple syrup, vanilla extract, and a pinch of salt.
2. Stir well to ensure all ingredients are evenly mixed.
3. Cover the jar or container and refrigerate overnight or for at least 4

hours.

4. In the morning, give the mixture a good stir and add your favorite toppings such as fresh berries, sliced bananas, nuts, or a drizzle of additional honey.

5. Enjoy a nutritious and delicious breakfast with these classic overnight oats!

Spinach and Feta Egg Muffins

Ingredients:

- 6 large eggs
- 1 cup fresh spinach, chopped
- 1/2 cup feta cheese, crumbled
- 1/4 cup red bell pepper, diced
- 1/4 cup onion, finely chopped
- Salt and pepper to taste
- Cooking spray or olive oil for greasing

Preparation:

1. Preheat your oven to 350°F (175°C) and grease a muffin tin with cooking spray or a light coating of olive oil.
2. In a mixing bowl, whisk together the eggs and season with salt and pepper.
3. Add the chopped spinach, crumbled feta, diced red bell pepper, and finely chopped onion to the eggs. Mix well.
4. Pour the egg mixture evenly into each muffin cup.
5. Bake for 20-25 minutes or until the egg muffins are set and the tops are

lightly golden.

6. Allow the muffins to cool for a few minutes before removing them from the tin. Enjoy!

Quinoa Breakfast Bowl

Ingredients:

- 1 cup cooked quinoa
- 1/2 cup Greek yogurt
- 1/2 cup fresh berries (e.g., strawberries, blueberries, raspberries)
- 1 tablespoon honey or maple syrup
- 1/4 cup almonds, chopped
- 1/2 teaspoon vanilla extract

Preparation:

1. In a bowl, combine the cooked quinoa and Greek yogurt.
2. Top with fresh berries, chopped almonds, a drizzle of honey or maple syrup, and vanilla extract.
3. Mix well and savor this protein-packed and nutritious quinoa breakfast bowl.

Smashed Avocado on Whole-Grain Toast with Cherry Tomatoes

Ingredients:

- 1 ripe avocado
- 2 slices whole-grain bread, toasted
- Cherry tomatoes, halved
- Salt and pepper to taste
- Optional: Red pepper flakes
- Lemon wedges for serving

Preparation:

1. Scoop the avocado into a bowl and mash it with a fork.
2. Season the mashed avocado with salt and pepper.
3. Spread the smashed avocado evenly onto the toasted whole-grain bread slices.
4. Top with halved cherry tomatoes and, if desired, sprinkle with red pepper flakes.
5. Serve with lemon wedges for an extra burst of freshness.

Blueberry and Almond Butter Smoothie

Ingredients:

- 1 cup blueberries (fresh or frozen)
- 1 banana

- 1 tablespoon almond butter
- 1/2 cup Greek yogurt
- 1 cup almond milk
- Optional: Ice cubes

Preparation:

1. Place blueberries, banana, almond butter, Greek yogurt, and almond milk in a blender.
2. Blend until smooth and creamy.
3. Add ice cubes if desired and blend again.
4. Pour into a glass and enjoy this refreshing and protein-rich blueberry and almond butter smoothie.

Sweet Potato Hash with Eggs

Ingredients:

- 2 medium sweet potatoes, peeled and diced
- 1 bell pepper, diced
- 1 onion, diced
- 2 tablespoons olive oil
- 1 teaspoon smoked paprika
- 1/2 teaspoon cumin
- Salt and pepper to taste
- Eggs (as many as desired)
- Fresh cilantro or parsley for garnish

Preparation:

1. Heat olive oil in a skillet over medium heat.
2. Add diced sweet potatoes, bell pepper, and onion to the skillet.
3. Season with smoked paprika, cumin, salt, and pepper. Cook until sweet potatoes are tender.
4. Create wells in the hash and crack eggs into them.
5. Cover the skillet and cook until the eggs are done to your liking.
6. Garnish with fresh cilantro or parsley and serve this hearty sweet potato hash with eggs.

Banana Walnut Pancakes

Ingredients:

- 1 cup all-purpose flour
- 1 tablespoon sugar
- 1 teaspoon baking powder
- 1/2 teaspoon baking soda
- 1/4 teaspoon salt
- 1 cup buttermilk
- 1 ripe banana, mashed
- 1/2 cup chopped walnuts
- 1 large egg
- 2 tablespoons unsalted butter, melted
- Maple syrup for serving

Preparation:

1. In a bowl, whisk together the flour, sugar, baking powder, baking soda, and salt.
2. In another bowl, mix buttermilk, mashed banana, chopped walnuts, egg, and melted butter.
3. Combine the wet and dry ingredients, stirring until just combined.
4. Heat a griddle or skillet over medium heat and lightly grease with butter or cooking spray.
5. Pour 1/4 cup of batter onto the griddle for each pancake.
6. Cook until bubbles form on the surface, then flip and cook until golden brown.
7. Serve the pancakes with maple syrup and extra banana slices if desired.

Apple Cinnamon Chia Pudding

Ingredients:

- 1/4 cup chia seeds
- 1 cup almond milk (or any preferred milk)
- 1 tablespoon maple syrup
- 1/2 teaspoon vanilla extract
- 1/2 teaspoon ground cinnamon
- 1 apple, diced
- Granola for topping (optional)

Preparation:

1. In a bowl, mix chia seeds, almond milk, maple syrup, vanilla extract, and ground cinnamon.
2. Stir well and refrigerate for at least 4 hours or overnight until the chia

seeds absorb the liquid.

3. Before serving, stir the chia pudding to ensure a smooth consistency.
4. Layer the chia pudding with diced apples in serving bowls or jars.
5. Top with granola for added crunch if desired.

Veggie and Hummus Breakfast Wrap

Ingredients:

- 1 whole-grain or spinach tortilla
- 2 tablespoons hummus
- 1/2 cup mixed veggies (e.g., bell peppers, cucumber, cherry tomatoes)
- 1/4 cup feta cheese, crumbled
- Fresh herbs (e.g., cilantro or parsley), chopped
- Salt and pepper to taste

Preparation:

1. Spread hummus evenly on the tortilla.
2. Arrange the mixed veggies on top of the hummus.
3. Sprinkle crumbled feta cheese and fresh herbs over the veggies.
4. Season with salt and pepper to taste.
5. Roll the tortilla tightly to form a wrap.
6. Slice in half diagonally and enjoy this nutritious and flavorful breakfast wrap.

Pomegranate and Pistachio Yogurt Parfait

Ingredients:

- 1 cup Greek yogurt
- 1/2 cup pomegranate arils
- 1/4 cup pistachios, chopped
- 1 tablespoon honey
- Granola for layering (optional)

Preparation:

1. In a glass or bowl, layer Greek yogurt at the bottom.
2. Add a layer of pomegranate arils.
3. Sprinkle chopped pistachios over the pomegranate layer.
4. Drizzle honey on top for sweetness.
5. Repeat the layers until the glass or bowl is filled.
6. Optionally, add a layer of granola for additional texture.
7. Serve and enjoy this delightful and nutrient-rich yogurt parfait.

Salmon and Avocado Bagel

Ingredients:

- 1 whole-grain bagel, sliced and toasted
- 4 ounces smoked salmon
- 1/2 avocado, sliced
- Cream cheese for spreading

- Fresh dill for garnish
- Lemon wedges for serving

Preparation:

1. Spread cream cheese on each half of the toasted bagel.
2. Layer smoked salmon over the cream cheese.
3. Top with slices of ripe avocado.
4. Garnish with fresh dill.
5. Serve with lemon wedges for a citrusy kick.
6. Enjoy this sophisticated and satisfying salmon and avocado bagel.

Coconut and Mango Chia Seed Smoothie Bowl

Ingredients:

- 1 cup frozen mango chunks
- 1/2 cup coconut milk
- 2 tablespoons chia seeds
- 1 tablespoon shredded coconut
- Fresh mango slices, granola, and mint for topping

Preparation:

1. In a blender, combine frozen mango chunks and coconut milk.
2. Blend until smooth and creamy.
3. Stir in chia seeds and shredded coconut.
4. Pour the smoothie into a bowl.

5. Top with fresh mango slices, granola, and a sprig of mint.
6. Enjoy this tropical and nutritious chia seed smoothie bowl.

Tomato Basil Mozzarella Frittata

Ingredients:

- 6 large eggs
- 1/4 cup milk
- 1 cup cherry tomatoes, halved
- 1/2 cup fresh mozzarella, diced
- 1/4 cup fresh basil, chopped
- Salt and pepper to taste
- Olive oil for greasing

Preparation:

1. Preheat your oven to 350°F (175°C).
2. In a bowl, whisk together eggs and milk.
3. Grease a baking dish with olive oil.
4. Pour the egg mixture into the baking dish.
5. Scatter cherry tomatoes, mozzarella, and fresh basil evenly.
6. Season with salt and pepper.
7. Bake for 20-25 minutes or until the frittata is set and golden.
8. Slice and serve this flavorful tomato basil mozzarella frittata.

Almond Butter Banana Toast

Ingredients:

- 2 slices whole-grain bread, toasted
- 2 tablespoons almond butter
- 1 banana, sliced
- Drizzle of honey
- Pinch of cinnamon (optional)

Preparation:

1. Spread almond butter evenly on each slice of toasted bread.
2. Arrange banana slices on top of the almond butter.
3. Drizzle with honey and sprinkle with cinnamon if desired.
4. Serve and savor this simple yet satisfying almond butter banana toast.

Mediterranean Breakfast Bowl

Ingredients:

- 1 cup cooked quinoa
- 1/2 cup cherry tomatoes, halved
- 1/4 cup cucumber, diced
- 2 tablespoons Kalamata olives, sliced
- 2 tablespoons feta cheese, crumbled
- Fresh parsley, chopped
- Olive oil and lemon juice for dressing

Preparation:

1. In a bowl, layer cooked quinoa.
2. Top with cherry tomatoes, diced cucumber, sliced Kalamata olives, and crumbled feta.
3. Sprinkle fresh parsley over the ingredients.
4. Drizzle with olive oil and lemon juice for a Mediterranean-inspired dressing.
5. Toss gently and enjoy this nutritious and flavorful breakfast bowl.

Chapter 5: Nourishing Lunches

Grilled Chicken Salad with Mixed Greens

Ingredients:

- Grilled chicken breast, sliced
- Mixed salad greens (lettuce, spinach, arugula)
- Cherry tomatoes, halved
- Cucumber, sliced
- Red onion, thinly sliced
- Balsamic vinaigrette dressing

Preparation:

1. Arrange the mixed salad greens on a plate.
2. Top with sliced grilled chicken, cherry tomatoes, cucumber, and red onion.
3. Drizzle with balsamic vinaigrette dressing.
4. Toss gently to combine and enjoy this satisfying grilled chicken salad.

Quinoa and Black Bean Bowl

Ingredients:

- Cooked quinoa
- Black beans, drained and rinsed
- Corn kernels, cooked
- Avocado, diced
- Red bell pepper, diced
- Lime vinaigrette dressing

Preparation:

1. In a bowl, combine cooked quinoa, black beans, corn, avocado, and red bell pepper.
2. Drizzle with lime vinaigrette dressing.
3. Toss the ingredients together and relish this nutritious quinoa and black bean bowl.

Mediterranean Chickpea Wrap

Ingredients:

- Whole wheat wrap
- Chickpeas, cooked and mashed
- Cucumber, diced
- Cherry tomatoes, halved
- Red onion, finely chopped

- Kalamata olives, sliced
- Feta cheese, crumbled
- Greek yogurt tzatziki sauce

Preparation:

1. Lay out the whole wheat wrap.
2. Spread mashed chickpeas over the wrap.
3. Add cucumber, cherry tomatoes, red onion, Kalamata olives, and crumbled feta.
4. Drizzle with Greek yogurt tzatziki sauce.
5. Fold the sides and roll the wrap, securing it with parchment paper if needed.
6. Enjoy this Mediterranean chickpea wrap as a flavorful and wholesome lunch.

Salmon and Quinoa Stuffed Bell Peppers

Ingredients:

- Bell peppers, halved and seeds removed
- Cooked quinoa
- Grilled salmon, flaked
- Spinach, chopped
- Feta cheese, crumbled
- Lemon dill sauce

Preparation:

1. Preheat the oven to 375°F (190°C).
2. In a bowl, mix cooked quinoa, grilled salmon, chopped spinach, and crumbled feta.
3. Stuff the bell peppers with the quinoa and salmon mixture.
4. Bake in the oven for 20-25 minutes or until the peppers are tender.
5. Drizzle with lemon dill sauce before serving these salmon and quinoa stuffed bell peppers.

Vegetarian Buddha Bowl

Ingredients:

- Brown rice, cooked
- Chickpeas, roasted
- Sweet potato, roasted and diced
- Broccoli, steamed
- Avocado, sliced
- Tahini dressing

Preparation:

1. Arrange brown rice as the base in a bowl.
2. Add roasted chickpeas, diced sweet potato, steamed broccoli, and sliced avocado.
3. Drizzle with tahini dressing.
4. Mix the ingredients together and savor the flavors of this nourishing vegetarian Buddha bowl.

Caprese Avocado Toast

Ingredients:

- Whole-grain bread, toasted
- Ripe avocado, mashed
- Tomato, sliced
- Fresh mozzarella, sliced
- Basil leaves
- Balsamic glaze

Preparation:

- Spread mashed avocado on toasted whole-grain bread.
- Top with tomato slices, fresh mozzarella, and basil leaves.
- Drizzle with balsamic glaze.
- Enjoy this delightful Caprese avocado toast for a light and tasty lunch.
- These lunch options offer a variety of flavors and nutrients to keep you satisfied and energized throughout the day.

Turkey and Veggie Lettuce Wraps

Ingredients:

- Ground turkey
- Lettuce leaves (such as iceberg or butter lettuce)
- Bell peppers, diced
- Carrots, shredded

- Green onions, sliced
- Hoisin sauce
- Soy sauce
- Sesame oil
- Sriracha (optional)

Preparation:

1. In a skillet, cook ground turkey until browned.
2. Add diced bell peppers, shredded carrots, and sliced green onions.
3. Stir in hoisin sauce, soy sauce, sesame oil, and sriracha if desired.
4. Spoon the turkey and veggie mixture onto lettuce leaves.
5. Roll the lettuce leaves to create wraps.
6. Enjoy these flavorful and low-carb turkey and veggie lettuce wraps.

Whole Wheat Veggie Pasta Salad

Ingredients:

- Whole wheat pasta, cooked
- Cherry tomatoes, halved
- Cucumber, diced
- Bell peppers, diced
- Red onion, finely chopped
- Kalamata olives, sliced
- Feta cheese, crumbled
- Olive oil and balsamic vinegar dressing

Preparation:

1. In a large bowl, combine cooked whole wheat pasta, cherry tomatoes, cucumber, bell peppers, red onion, Kalamata olives, and crumbled feta.
2. Drizzle with olive oil and balsamic vinegar dressing.
3. Toss the ingredients together and chill before serving.
4. Enjoy this wholesome and satisfying whole wheat veggie pasta salad.

Sweet Potato and Black Bean Quesadilla

Ingredients:

- Whole wheat tortillas
- Sweet potatoes, roasted and mashed
- Black beans, cooked and mashed
- Red onion, finely chopped
- Cilantro, chopped
- Shredded cheddar cheese
- Avocado slices (optional)

Preparation:

1. Spread mashed sweet potatoes on one half of a whole wheat tortilla.
2. Top with mashed black beans, chopped red onion, cilantro, and shredded cheddar cheese.
3. Fold the tortilla in half.
4. Cook in a skillet until the cheese is melted and the tortilla is golden brown.
5. Slice and serve with optional avocado slices.

6. Enjoy these flavorful sweet potato and black bean quesadillas.

Greek Quinoa Salad with Grilled Shrimp

Ingredients:

- Quinoa, cooked
- Grilled shrimp
- Cherry tomatoes, halved
- Cucumber, diced
- Red onion, finely chopped
- Feta cheese, crumbled
- Kalamata olives, sliced
- Greek dressing

Preparation:

1. In a bowl, combine cooked quinoa, grilled shrimp, cherry tomatoes, cucumber, red onion, crumbled feta, and sliced Kalamata olives.
2. Drizzle with Greek dressing.
3. Toss the ingredients together and enjoy this protein-packed Greek quinoa salad.

Chickpea and Vegetable Stir-Fry

Ingredients:

- Chickpeas, cooked
- Mixed vegetables (broccoli, bell peppers, snap peas, carrots), sliced
- Garlic, minced
- Soy sauce
- Sesame oil
- Ginger, grated
- Red pepper flakes (optional)
- Green onions, sliced

Preparation:

1. In a wok or skillet, stir-fry chickpeas and mixed vegetables with garlic.
2. Add soy sauce, sesame oil, grated ginger, and red pepper flakes if desired.
3. Continue to stir-fry until the vegetables are tender-crisp.
4. Garnish with sliced green onions.
5. Serve this flavorful chickpea and vegetable stir-fry over rice or noodles.

Roasted Vegetable and Hummus Wrap

Ingredients:

- Whole wheat wrap
- Roasted vegetables (zucchini, bell peppers, eggplant, cherry tomatoes)
- Hummus

- Spinach leaves
- Feta cheese, crumbled

Preparation:

1. Lay out the whole wheat wrap.
2. Spread hummus over the wrap.
3. Arrange roasted vegetables, spinach leaves, and crumbled feta.
4. Fold the sides and roll the wrap, securing it with parchment paper if needed.
5. Enjoy this nutritious and tasty roasted vegetable and hummus wrap.

Tuna and White Bean Salad

Ingredients:

- Canned tuna, drained
- White beans, drained and rinsed
- Cherry tomatoes, halved
- Red onion, finely chopped
- Cucumber, diced
- Kalamata olives, sliced
- Fresh parsley, chopped
- Olive oil and lemon dressing

Preparation:

1. In a bowl, combine canned tuna, white beans, cherry tomatoes, red

onion, cucumber, Kalamata olives, and fresh parsley.

2. Drizzle with olive oil and lemon dressing.
3. Toss the ingredients gently to coat them in the dressing.
4. Chill before serving and enjoy this protein-rich tuna and white bean salad.

Cauliflower Rice Bowl with Teriyaki Tofu

Ingredients:

- Cauliflower rice, cooked
- Extra-firm tofu, cubed and sautéed in teriyaki sauce
- Broccoli florets, steamed
- Carrots, julienned and sautéed
- Edamame, steamed
- Green onions, sliced
- Sesame seeds
- Teriyaki sauce

Preparation:

1. Cook cauliflower rice according to package instructions.
2. Sauté cubed tofu in teriyaki sauce until golden brown.
3. Assemble the bowl with cauliflower rice, teriyaki tofu, steamed broccoli, sautéed carrots, and edamame.
4. Garnish with sliced green onions and sesame seeds.
5. Drizzle with additional teriyaki sauce if desired.
6. Enjoy this flavorful and low-carb cauliflower rice bowl with teriyaki tofu.

Pesto Chicken Quinoa Bowl

Ingredients:

- Quinoa, cooked
- Grilled chicken breast, sliced
- Cherry tomatoes, halved
- Avocado, sliced
- Pesto sauce
- Pine nuts, toasted
- Fresh basil leaves

Preparation:

1. In a bowl, arrange cooked quinoa, grilled chicken breast slices, cherry tomatoes, and avocado.
2. Drizzle with pesto sauce.
3. Sprinkle toasted pine nuts over the bowl.
4. Garnish with fresh basil leaves.
5. Toss the ingredients gently to combine the flavors.
6. Savor this delightful and protein-packed pesto chicken quinoa bowl.

Chapter 6: Wholesome Dinners

Baked Lemon Herb Chicken with Roasted Vegetables

Ingredients:

- Chicken breasts, boneless and skinless
- Lemon juice
- Olive oil
- Garlic, minced
- Fresh herbs (rosemary, thyme, oregano), chopped
- Salt and pepper to taste
- Assorted vegetables (carrots, potatoes, Brussels sprouts), chopped

Preparation:

1. Preheat the oven to 375°F (190°C).
2. In a bowl, mix lemon juice, olive oil, minced garlic, chopped herbs, salt, and pepper.
3. Place chicken breasts and assorted vegetables in a baking dish.
4. Pour the lemon herb mixture over the chicken and vegetables.
5. Bake in the oven for 25-30 minutes or until the chicken is cooked

through and vegetables are tender.

6. Serve this baked lemon herb chicken with roasted vegetables for a wholesome dinner.

Lentil and Vegetable Curry with Brown Rice

Ingredients:

- Brown lentils, cooked
- Mixed vegetables (bell peppers, peas, carrots, spinach)
- Onion, finely chopped
- Garlic, minced
- Ginger, grated
- Curry powder
- Coconut milk
- Tomato sauce
- Brown rice, cooked

Preparation:

1. In a pot, sauté chopped onion, minced garlic, and grated ginger until fragrant.
2. Add mixed vegetables and cook until slightly tender.
3. Stir in cooked brown lentils, curry powder, coconut milk, and tomato sauce.
4. Simmer until the vegetables are cooked through and the curry has thickened.
5. Serve over cooked brown rice for a delicious and hearty lentil and vegetable curry.

Grilled Salmon with Quinoa and Asparagus

Ingredients:

- Salmon fillets
- Lemon zest
- Olive oil
- Salt and pepper to taste
- Quinoa, cooked
- Asparagus spears, trimmed
- Lemon wedges for garnish

Preparation:

1. Preheat the grill to medium-high heat.
2. Brush salmon fillets with olive oil, sprinkle with lemon zest, salt, and pepper.
3. Grill salmon for 4-5 minutes per side or until cooked to your liking.
4. Grill asparagus until tender.
5. Serve grilled salmon over cooked quinoa with grilled asparagus on the side.
6. Garnish with lemon wedges and enjoy this healthy and flavorful dish.
7.

Spinach and Feta Stuffed Chicken Breast with Sweet Potato Mash

Ingredients:

- Chicken breasts, boneless and skinless
- Fresh spinach leaves
- Feta cheese, crumbled
- Garlic, minced
- Sweet potatoes, peeled, diced, and boiled
- Butter
- Milk
- Salt and pepper to taste

Preparation:

1. Preheat the oven to 375°F (190°C).
2. Cut a pocket into each chicken breast.
3. Stuff the pockets with fresh spinach and crumbled feta.
4. Season chicken breasts with minced garlic, salt, and pepper.
5. Bake in the oven for 25-30 minutes or until chicken is cooked through.
6. Mash boiled sweet potatoes with butter, milk, salt, and pepper.
7. Serve spinach and feta stuffed chicken breast over sweet potato mash.

Chickpea and Spinach Stew over Couscous

Ingredients:

- Chickpeas, cooked
- Fresh spinach leaves
- Onion, finely chopped
- Garlic, minced
- Vegetable broth
- Tomatoes, diced
- Ground cumin
- Ground coriander
- Paprika
- Couscous, cooked

Preparation:

1. In a pot, sauté chopped onion and minced garlic until softened.
2. Add chickpeas, fresh spinach, diced tomatoes, ground cumin, ground coriander, paprika, and vegetable broth.
3. Simmer until spinach wilts and flavors meld.
4. Serve this hearty chickpea and spinach stew over cooked couscous.

Teriyaki Tofu Stir-Fry with Broccoli and Brown Rice

Ingredients:

- Extra-firm tofu, cubed
- Broccoli florets
- Brown rice, cooked
- Teriyaki sauce
- Soy sauce
- Sesame oil

- Garlic, minced
- Ginger, grated
- Green onions, sliced

Preparation:

1. Sauté cubed tofu in sesame oil until golden brown.
2. Add broccoli florets, minced garlic, and grated ginger.
3. Pour teriyaki sauce and soy sauce over the tofu and broccoli.
4. Stir-fry until broccoli is tender-crisp.
5. Serve over cooked brown rice and garnish with sliced green onions.

Mediterranean Baked Cod with Tomato and Olive Relish

Ingredients:

- Cod fillets
- Cherry tomatoes, halved
- Kalamata olives, sliced
- Red onion, finely chopped
- Garlic, minced
- Olive oil
- Lemon juice
- Fresh basil, chopped
- Salt and pepper to taste

Preparation:

1. Preheat the oven to 400°F (200°C).
2. Place cod fillets in a baking dish.
3. In a bowl, mix cherry tomatoes, Kalamata olives, red onion, minced garlic, olive oil, lemon juice, fresh basil, salt, and pepper.
4. Spoon the tomato and olive relish over the cod fillets.
5. Bake in the oven for 15-20 minutes or until the cod is cooked through.
6. Serve this Mediterranean baked cod with a flavorful tomato and olive relish.

Quinoa and Black Bean Stuffed Peppers

Ingredients:

- Bell peppers, halved and seeds removed
- Quinoa, cooked
- Black beans, cooked
- Corn kernels
- Red onion, diced
- Tomatoes, diced
- Mexican seasoning
- Shredded cheese (cheddar or Mexican blend)
- Fresh cilantro, chopped

Preparation:

1. Preheat the oven to 375°F (190°C).
2. In a bowl, mix cooked quinoa, black beans, corn, red onion, diced tomatoes, and Mexican seasoning.
3. Stuff the halved bell peppers with the quinoa and black bean mixture.

4. Top each stuffed pepper with shredded cheese.
5. Bake in the oven for 20-25 minutes or until the peppers are tender.
6. Garnish with chopped cilantro before serving.

Shrimp and Avocado Salad with Citrus Vinaigrette

Ingredients:

- Shrimp, peeled and deveined
- Mixed salad greens
- Avocado, sliced
- Grapefruit segments
- Orange segments
- Red onion, thinly sliced
- Cherry tomatoes, halved
- Olive oil
- Lemon juice
- Dijon mustard
- Honey
- Salt and pepper to taste

Preparation:

1. Cook shrimp in a pan until pink and opaque.
2. In a large bowl, combine salad greens, sliced avocado, grapefruit segments, orange segments, sliced red onion, and cherry tomatoes.
3. In a separate bowl, whisk together olive oil, lemon juice, Dijon mustard, honey, salt, and pepper to make the citrus vinaigrette.
4. Toss the salad with the citrus vinaigrette.

5. Top the salad with cooked shrimp and serve.

Butternut Squash and Kale Risotto

Ingredients:

- Arborio rice
- Butternut squash, diced
- Kale, chopped
- Onion, finely chopped
- Garlic, minced
- Vegetable broth
- White wine
- Parmesan cheese, grated
- Butter
- Olive oil
- Salt and pepper to taste

Preparation:

1. In a large pan, sauté chopped onion and minced garlic in olive oil until softened.
2. Add Arborio rice and cook until lightly toasted.
3. Pour in white wine and cook until mostly evaporated.
4. Begin adding vegetable broth gradually, stirring frequently until the rice is creamy and cooked al dente.
5. In the last few minutes of cooking, stir in diced butternut squash and chopped kale.
6. Remove from heat and stir in grated Parmesan cheese and butter.

7. Season with salt and pepper to taste before serving.

Turkey and Vegetable Skewers with Quinoa Pilaf

Ingredients:

- Turkey breast, cut into cubes
- Bell peppers, cut into chunks
- Zucchini, sliced
- Cherry tomatoes
- Red onion, cut into wedges
- Quinoa, cooked
- Lemon zest
- Fresh parsley, chopped
- Olive oil
- Garlic powder
- Paprika
- Salt and pepper to taste

Preparation:

1. Preheat the grill or grill pan.
2. Thread turkey cubes, bell peppers, zucchini, cherry tomatoes, and red onion onto skewers.
3. In a bowl, mix cooked quinoa with lemon zest, chopped fresh parsley, olive oil, garlic powder, paprika, salt, and pepper to make the quinoa pilaf.
4. Grill the skewers until the turkey is cooked through and vegetables are charred.

5. Serve the turkey and vegetable skewers over the quinoa pilaf.

Eggplant Parmesan with Whole Wheat Spaghetti

Ingredients:

- Eggplant, sliced
- Whole wheat spaghetti, cooked
- Marinara sauce
- Mozzarella cheese, shredded
- Parmesan cheese, grated
- Fresh basil leaves
- Olive oil
- Salt and pepper to taste

Preparation:

1. Preheat the oven to 375°F (190°C).
2. Coat eggplant slices with olive oil, salt, and pepper, then bake until tender.
3. In a baking dish, layer cooked whole wheat spaghetti, marinara sauce, baked eggplant slices, and shredded mozzarella.
4. Repeat the layers, finishing with a layer of mozzarella and grated Parmesan.
5. Bake until the cheese is melted and bubbly.
6. Garnish with fresh basil leaves before serving.

Balsamic Glazed Chicken Thighs with Brussels Sprouts

Ingredients:

- Chicken thighs, bone-in and skin-on
- Brussels sprouts, halved
- Balsamic vinegar
- Honey
- Dijon mustard
- Garlic, minced
- Olive oil
- Salt and pepper to taste

Preparation:

1. Preheat the oven to 400°F (200°C).
2. In a bowl, whisk together balsamic vinegar, honey, Dijon mustard, minced garlic, olive oil, salt, and pepper.
3. Place chicken thighs and Brussels sprouts on a baking sheet.
4. Brush the balsamic glaze over the chicken and Brussels sprouts.
5. Bake in the oven until the chicken is cooked through and Brussels sprouts are caramelized.
6. Serve the balsamic glazed chicken thighs with roasted Brussels sprouts.

Zucchini Noodles with Pesto and Cherry Tomatoes

Ingredients:

- Zucchini, spiralized into noodles
- Cherry tomatoes, halved
- Pesto sauce
- Pine nuts, toasted
- Parmesan cheese, grated
- Olive oil
- Salt and pepper to taste

Preparation:

1. In a pan, sauté zucchini noodles in olive oil until just tender.
2. Toss the zucchini noodles with pesto sauce and cherry tomatoes.
3. Sprinkle with toasted pine nuts and grated Parmesan.
4. Season with salt and pepper to taste.
5. Serve this light and flavorful zucchini noodle dish.

Beef and Vegetable Stir-Fry with Cauliflower Rice

Ingredients:

- Beef sirloin, thinly sliced
- Broccoli florets
- Bell peppers, sliced
- Carrots, julienned
- Snap peas
- Cauliflower rice, cooked
- Soy sauce
- Sesame oil
- Ginger, grated

- Garlic, minced
- Green onions, sliced

Preparation:

1. In a wok or skillet, stir-fry thinly sliced beef until browned.
2. Add broccoli florets, sliced bell peppers, julienned carrots, and snap peas.
3. In a small bowl, mix soy sauce, sesame oil, grated ginger, and minced garlic.
4. Pour the sauce over the beef and vegetables and stir-fry until everything is cooked.
5. Serve the beef and vegetable stir-fry over cooked cauliflower rice.
6. Garnish with sliced green onions before serving.

Chapter 7: Sides and Snacks

Roasted Garlic Hummus with Veggie Sticks

Ingredients:

- Store-bought or homemade roasted garlic hummus
- Assorted veggie sticks (carrots, cucumber, bell peppers)

Preparation:

1. Arrange the veggie sticks on a serving platter.
2. Place a bowl of roasted garlic hummus in the center.
3. Dip the veggie sticks into the hummus and enjoy this wholesome and flavorful snack.

Baked Sweet Potato Fries

Ingredients:

- Sweet potatoes, cut into fries
- Olive oil
- Paprika, garlic powder, and salt to taste
- Fresh parsley, chopped (optional, for garnish)

Preparation:

1. Preheat the oven to 425°F (220°C).
2. Toss sweet potato fries with olive oil, paprika, garlic powder, and salt.
3. Spread the fries in a single layer on a baking sheet.
4. Bake for 20-25 minutes or until crispy and golden.
5. Garnish with chopped fresh parsley if desired.
6. Serve these baked sweet potato fries as a delightful and healthier alternative to traditional fries.

Caprese Skewers

Ingredients:

- Cherry tomatoes
- Fresh mozzarella balls
- Fresh basil leaves
- Balsamic glaze for drizzling

Preparation:

1. Thread a cherry tomato, a fresh mozzarella ball, and a fresh basil leaf onto small skewers.
2. Arrange the skewers on a serving platter.
3. Drizzle with balsamic glaze just before serving.
4. Enjoy these easy and elegant caprese skewers as a tasty snack or side dish.

Guacamole with Whole Grain Tortilla Chips

Ingredients:

- Ripe avocados, mashed
- Tomato, diced
- Red onion, finely chopped
- Garlic, minced
- Lime juice
- Fresh cilantro, chopped
- Salt and pepper to taste
- Whole grain tortilla chips for dipping

Preparation:

1. In a bowl, combine mashed avocados, diced tomato, finely chopped red onion, minced garlic, lime juice, and chopped fresh cilantro.
2. Season with salt and pepper to taste.
3. Serve with whole-grain tortilla chips for a nutritious and satisfying guacamole dip.

Cucumber and Greek Yogurt Dip

Ingredients:

- Greek yogurt
- Cucumber, grated and drained
- Garlic, minced
- Dill, chopped
- Lemon juice
- Salt and pepper to taste

Preparation:

1. In a bowl, mix Greek yogurt with grated and drained cucumber, minced garlic, chopped dill, and a splash of lemon juice.
2. Season with salt and pepper to taste.
3. Refrigerate for at least 30 minutes before serving.
4. Enjoy this refreshing and creamy cucumber and Greek yogurt dip with your favorite veggies or whole-grain crackers.

Quinoa-Stuffed Mushrooms

Ingredients:

- Large mushroom stems removed
- Quinoa, cooked
- Spinach, chopped
- Feta cheese, crumbled

- Garlic, minced
- Olive oil
- Salt and pepper to taste

Preparation:

1. Preheat the oven to 375°F (190°C).
2. In a bowl, mix cooked quinoa with chopped spinach, crumbled feta cheese, minced garlic, and a drizzle of olive oil.
3. Season with salt and pepper to taste.
4. Stuff the mushrooms with the quinoa mixture.
5. Bake for 15-20 minutes or until the mushrooms are tender.
6. Serve these quinoa-stuffed mushrooms as a flavorful and nutritious side or snack.

Cheese and Whole Wheat Crackers Platter

Ingredients:

- Assorted cheeses (cheddar, brie, gouda, etc.), sliced
- Whole wheat crackers
- Grapes or apple slices (optional, for garnish)

Preparation:

1. Arrange the sliced cheeses and whole wheat crackers on a serving platter.
2. Add grapes or apple slices for a touch of sweetness if desired.
3. Serve this cheese and whole wheat crackers platter as an easy and elegant

appetizer or snack.

Roasted Chickpeas

Ingredients:

- Canned chickpeas, drained and rinsed
- Olive oil
- Smoked paprika, cumin, and garlic powder to taste
- Salt and pepper to taste

Preparation:

1. Preheat the oven to 400°F (200°C).
2. Pat dry the chickpeas with a paper towel to remove excess moisture.
3. Toss chickpeas with olive oil, smoked paprika, cumin, garlic powder, salt, and pepper.
4. Spread the chickpeas on a baking sheet in a single layer.
5. Roast for 25-30 minutes or until crispy.
6. Allow cooling before serving these flavorful roasted chickpeas as a crunchy snack.

Greek Salad Skewers

Ingredients:

- Cherry tomatoes
- Cucumber, diced
- Kalamata olives, pitted
- Feta cheese, cubed
- Red onion, finely chopped
- Greek dressing for drizzling

Preparation:

1. Thread a cherry tomato, a cube of feta, a piece of cucumber, a Kalamata olive, and a sprinkle of finely chopped red onion onto small skewers.
2. Arrange the skewers on a serving platter.
3. Drizzle with Greek dressing just before serving.
4. Enjoy these delightful Greek salad skewers as a light and refreshing appetizer.

Veggie Spring Rolls with Peanut Dipping Sauce

Ingredients:

- Rice paper wrappers
- Shredded cabbage
- Carrots, julienned
- Cucumber, julienned
- Avocado, sliced
- Fresh mint leaves
- Rice vermicelli noodles, cooked and cooled
- Peanut dipping sauce (store-bought or homemade)

Preparation:

1. Dip a rice paper wrapper in warm water for a few seconds until it softens.
2. Lay the wrapper on a flat surface and fill it with shredded cabbage, julienned carrots, julienned cucumber, avocado slices, fresh mint leaves, and cooked rice vermicelli noodles.
3. Fold the sides of the wrapper and roll it tightly.
4. Repeat with remaining ingredients.
5. Serve these veggie spring rolls with peanut dipping sauce for a light and flavorful snack or appetizer.

Baked Parmesan Zucchini Chips

Ingredients:

- Zucchini, thinly sliced
- Parmesan cheese, grated
- Olive oil
- Garlic powder, onion powder, and dried oregano to taste
- Salt and pepper to taste

Preparation:

1. Preheat the oven to 425°F (220°C).
2. Toss thinly sliced zucchini with olive oil, grated Parmesan cheese, garlic powder, onion powder, dried oregano, salt, and pepper.
3. Arrange the zucchini slices on a baking sheet in a single layer.
4. Bake for 15-20 minutes or until golden and crispy.
5. Let cool before serving these baked Parmesan zucchini chips as a tasty

and healthier alternative to traditional chips.

Mixed Berry Yogurt Parfait

Ingredients:

- Greek yogurt
- Mixed berries (strawberries, blueberries, raspberries)
- Granola
- Honey for drizzling (optional)

Preparation:

1. In a glass or bowl, layer Greek yogurt with mixed berries and granola.
2. Repeat the layers until the container is filled.
3. Drizzle with honey if desired.
4. Serve this mixed berry yogurt parfait as a delicious and nutritious snack or dessert.

Salsa and Black Bean Corn Cups

Ingredients:

- Black beans, cooked
- Corn kernels (fresh or thawed if frozen)
- Cherry tomatoes, diced

- Red onion, finely chopped
- Fresh cilantro, chopped
- Lime juice
- Salt and pepper to taste
- Tortilla cups or chips for serving

Preparation:

1. In a bowl, combine black beans, corn kernels, diced cherry tomatoes, finely chopped red onion, and chopped fresh cilantro.
2. Drizzle with lime juice and toss to combine.
3. Season with salt and pepper to taste.
4. Spoon the salsa into tortilla cups or serve with tortilla chips.
5. Enjoy these salsa and black bean corn cups as a flavorful and colorful appetizer.

Spicy Edamame

Ingredients:

- Edamame, cooked and shelled
- Sesame oil
- Soy sauce
- Sriracha or chili flakes to taste
- Sesame seeds for garnish (optional)

Preparation:

1. In a bowl, toss cooked and shelled edamame with sesame oil, soy sauce, and sriracha or chili flakes.
2. Mix until the edamame is well-coated with the spicy seasoning.
3. Garnish with sesame seeds if desired.
4. Serve this spicy edamame as a protein-packed and zesty snack.

Baba Ganoush with Pita Bread

Ingredients:

- Eggplants
- Garlic, minced
- Tahini
- Lemon juice
- Olive oil
- Salt and pepper to taste
- Pita bread for dipping

Preparation:

1. Roast or grill the eggplants until the skin is charred and the flesh is soft.
2. Allow the eggplants to cool, then peel off the skin.
3. In a blender or food processor, combine the eggplant flesh with minced garlic, tahini, lemon juice, olive oil, salt, and pepper.
4. Blend until smooth.
5. Transfer the baba ganoush to a serving bowl.
6. Serve with pita bread for a delicious and smoky dip.

Chapter 8: Desserts with a Heart-Healthy Twist

Dark Chocolate-Dipped Strawberries

Ingredients:

- Fresh strawberries, washed and dried
- Dark chocolate, melted

Preparation:

1. Dip each strawberry into the melted dark chocolate, ensuring it is well-coated.
2. Place the dipped strawberries on a parchment-lined tray.
3. Allow the chocolate to set in the refrigerator.
4. Enjoy these dark chocolate-dipped strawberries as a simple and decadent heart-healthy dessert.

Oatmeal Banana Cookies

Ingredients:

- Ripe bananas, mashed
- Rolled oats
- Cinnamon
- Vanilla extract
- Nuts or raisins (optional)

Preparation:

1. Preheat the oven to 350°F (180°C).
2. In a bowl, mix mashed ripe bananas with rolled oats, cinnamon, vanilla extract, and nuts or raisins if desired.
3. Drop spoonfuls of the mixture onto a baking sheet.
4. Bake for 12-15 minutes or until the edges are golden.
5. Allow to cool before enjoying these oatmeal banana cookies as a wholesome treat.

Greek Yogurt and Berry Popsicles

Ingredients:

- Greek yogurt
- Mixed berries (strawberries, blueberries, raspberries)
- Honey or maple syrup (optional)

Preparation:

1. In a blender, mix Greek yogurt with mixed berries and sweeten with honey or maple syrup if desired.
2. Pour the mixture into popsicle molds.
3. Insert popsicle sticks and freeze until solid.
4. Run the molds under warm water to release the popsicles.
5. Indulge in these refreshing Greek yogurt and berry popsicles for a guilt-free dessert.

Avocado Chocolate Mousse

Ingredients:

- Ripe avocados, peeled and pitted
- Cocoa powder
- Maple syrup or agave nectar
- Vanilla extract
- Almond milk

Preparation:

1. In a blender, combine ripe avocados, cocoa powder, maple syrup or agave nectar, vanilla extract, and a splash of almond milk.
2. Blend until smooth and creamy.
3. Chill the chocolate mousse in the refrigerator.
4. Serve this avocado chocolate mousse as a rich and satisfying heart-healthy dessert.

Almond Flour Blueberry Muffins

Ingredients:

- Almond flour
- Baking powder
- Eggs
- Almond milk
- Maple syrup
- Vanilla extract
- Fresh or frozen blueberries

Preparation:

1. Preheat the oven to 350°F (180°C) and line a muffin tin with paper liners.
2. In a bowl, mix almond flour with baking powder.
3. In another bowl, whisk eggs, almond milk, maple syrup, and vanilla extract.
4. Combine the wet and dry ingredients, then fold in the blueberries.
5. Spoon the batter into the muffin tin.
6. Bake for 20-25 minutes or until a toothpick comes out clean.
7. Allow to cool before enjoying these almond flour blueberry muffins as a delightful and nutty treat.

Dark Chocolate-Dipped Strawberries

Ingredients:

- Fresh strawberries, washed and dried
- Dark chocolate, melted

Preparation:

1. Dip each strawberry into the melted dark chocolate, ensuring it is well-coated.
2. Place the dipped strawberries on a parchment-lined tray.
3. Allow the chocolate to set in the refrigerator.
4. Enjoy these dark chocolate-dipped strawberries as a simple and decadent heart-healthy dessert.

Oatmeal Banana Cookies

Ingredients:

- Ripe bananas, mashed
- Rolled oats
- Cinnamon
- Vanilla extract
- Nuts or raisins (optional)

Preparation:

1. Preheat the oven to 350°F (180°C).
2. In a bowl, mix mashed ripe bananas with rolled oats, cinnamon, vanilla extract, and nuts or raisins if desired.
3. Drop spoonfuls of the mixture onto a baking sheet.

4. Bake for 12-15 minutes or until the edges are golden.
5. Allow to cool before enjoying these oatmeal banana cookies as a wholesome treat.

Greek Yogurt and Berry Popsicles

Ingredients:

- Greek yogurt
- Mixed berries (strawberries, blueberries, raspberries)
- Honey or maple syrup (optional)

Preparation:

1. In a blender, mix Greek yogurt with mixed berries and sweeten with honey or maple syrup if desired.
2. Pour the mixture into popsicle molds.
3. Insert popsicle sticks and freeze until solid.
4. Run the molds under warm water to release the popsicles.
5. Indulge in these refreshing Greek yogurt and berry popsicles for a guilt-free dessert.

Avocado Chocolate Mousse

Ingredients:

- Ripe avocados, peeled and pitted
- Cocoa powder
- Maple syrup or agave nectar
- Vanilla extract
- Almond milk

Preparation:

1. In a blender, combine ripe avocados, cocoa powder, maple syrup or agave nectar, vanilla extract, and a splash of almond milk.
2. Blend until smooth and creamy.
3. Chill the chocolate mousse in the refrigerator.
4. Serve this avocado chocolate mousse as a rich and satisfying heart-healthy dessert.

Almond Flour Blueberry Muffins

Ingredients:

- Almond flour
- Baking powder
- Eggs
- Almond milk
- Maple syrup
- Vanilla extract
- Fresh or frozen blueberries

Preparation:

1. Preheat the oven to 350°F (180°C) and line a muffin tin with paper liners.
2. In a bowl, mix almond flour with baking powder.
3. In another bowl, whisk eggs, almond milk, maple syrup, and vanilla extract.
4. Combine the wet and dry ingredients, then fold in the blueberries.
5. Spoon the batter into the muffin tin.
6. Bake for 20-25 minutes or until a toothpick comes out clean.
7. Allow to cool before enjoying these almond flour blueberry muffins as a delightful and nutty treat.

Mango Sorbet

Ingredients:

- Ripe mangoes, peeled and diced
- Lime juice
- Honey or agave syrup (optional)
- Fresh mint leaves for garnish (optional)

Preparation:

1. Place the diced mangoes in a blender or food processor.
2. Add lime juice and sweeten with honey or agave syrup if desired.
3. Blend until smooth.
4. Pour the mango mixture into a shallow dish and spread it evenly.
5. Freeze for at least 4 hours or until firm.
6. Before serving, let the sorbet sit at room temperature for a few minutes.
7. Scoop into bowls, garnish with fresh mint leaves if desired, and enjoy this refreshing mango sorbet.

Pecan and Date Energy Bites

Ingredients:

- Pecans
- Dates, pitted
- Rolled oats
- Chia seeds
- Vanilla extract
- Salt

Preparation:

1. In a food processor, combine pecans, dates, rolled oats, chia seeds, vanilla extract, and a pinch of salt.
2. Pulse until the mixture forms a sticky dough.
3. Scoop out small portions and roll them into bite-sized balls.
4. Place the energy bites on a parchment-lined tray.
5. Refrigerate for at least 30 minutes before serving.
6. Enjoy these pecan and date energy bites as a nutritious and satisfying snack.

Chapter 9: Beverages for Heart Health

Green Tea Infusion with Citrus Twist

Ingredients:

- Green tea bags
- Boiling water
- Orange slices
- Lemon slices
- Fresh mint leaves
- Honey or agave syrup (optional)

Preparation:

1. Place green tea bags in a teapot or heatproof pitcher.
2. Pour boiling water over the tea bags and let steep for 3-5 minutes.
3. Add orange slices, lemon slices, and fresh mint leaves to the tea.
4. Sweeten with honey or agave syrup if desired.
5. Allow the infusion to cool, then refrigerate.
6. Serve over ice and garnish with additional citrus slices and mint leaves.

Berry Blast Smoothie with Flaxseed

Ingredients:

- Mixed berries (strawberries, blueberries, raspberries)
- Greek yogurt
- Flaxseed
- Honey or maple syrup
- Almond milk
- Ice cubes

Preparation:

1. In a blender, combine mixed berries, Greek yogurt, flaxseed, honey or maple syrup, and almond milk.
2. Blend until smooth and creamy.
3. Add ice cubes and blend again until the smoothie reaches your desired consistency.
4. Pour into glasses and enjoy this nutritious berry blast smoothie.

Hibiscus and Ginger Iced Tea

Ingredients:

- Hibiscus tea bags
- Fresh ginger, sliced
- Boiling water
- Honey or agave syrup

- Lemon slices
- Ice cubes
- Fresh mint leaves for garnish

Preparation:

1. Place hibiscus tea bags and sliced fresh ginger in a heatproof pitcher.
2. Pour boiling water over the tea bags and ginger, letting it steep for 5-7 minutes.
3. Sweeten with honey or agave syrup to taste.
4. Allow the tea to cool, then refrigerate until chilled.
5. Serve over ice with lemon slices and garnish with fresh mint leaves.

Kale and Pineapple Detox Juice

Ingredients:

- Kale leaves, stems removed
- Pineapple chunks
- Cucumber, peeled
- Lemon, peeled
- Ginger, peeled
- Water

Preparation:

1. In a juicer, process kale leaves, pineapple chunks, cucumber, lemon, and ginger.

2. Add water to adjust the consistency if needed.

3. Strain the juice to remove the pulp if desired.

4. Pour into glasses and enjoy this refreshing and detoxifying kale and

pineapple juice.

Golden Turmeric Latte

Ingredients:

- Turmeric powder
- Cinnamon
- Ginger powder
- Black pepper
- Honey or maple syrup
- Almond milk
- Hot water

Preparation:

1. In a small saucepan, whisk together turmeric powder, cinnamon, ginger powder, black pepper, and honey or maple syrup with hot water.

2. Heat the mixture over low-medium heat until it simmers.

3. Add almond milk and continue to heat until hot but not boiling.

4. Pour into mugs and savor the warming flavors of this golden turmeric latte.

Watermelon Mint Refresher

Ingredients:

- Fresh watermelon chunks
- Fresh mint leaves
- Lime juice
- Agave syrup
- Sparkling water
- Ice cubes

Preparation:

1. In a blender, combine fresh watermelon chunks, mint leaves, lime juice, and agave syrup.
2. Blend until smooth.
3. Strain the mixture if you prefer a smoother texture.
4. In glasses, pour the watermelon mint blend over ice cubes.
5. Top with sparkling water for a fizzy finish.
6. Garnish with mint leaves and enjoy this hydrating watermelon mint refresher.

Blueberry and Almond Milk Protein Shake

Ingredients:

- Blueberries, fresh or frozen
- Almond milk
- Protein powder (vanilla or berry flavor)
- Greek yogurt

- Almond butter
- Ice cubes

Preparation:

1. In a blender, combine blueberries, almond milk, protein powder, Greek yogurt, almond butter, and ice cubes.
2. Blend until smooth and creamy.
3. Pour into a glass and enjoy this delicious blueberry and almond milk protein shake for a nutritious boost.

Cucumber Basil Sparkling Water

Ingredients:

- Cucumber slices
- Fresh basil leaves
- Sparkling water
- Ice cubes
- Lemon slices for garnish

Preparation:

1. In a glass, add cucumber slices and fresh basil leaves.
2. Fill the glass with sparkling water and ice cubes.
3. Stir gently to infuse the flavors.
4. Garnish with lemon slices.
5. Refresh yourself with this cucumber basil sparkling water.

Cranberry and Orange Zest Mocktail

Ingredients:

- Cranberry juice
- Orange zest
- Sparkling water
- Ice cubes
- Fresh cranberries for garnish (optional)

Preparation:

1. Fill a glass with cranberry juice and add orange zest.
2. Top with sparkling water and ice cubes.
3. Stir gently to combine the flavors.
4. Garnish with fresh cranberries if desired.
5. Sip on this refreshing cranberry and orange zest mocktail.

Matcha Green Tea Smoothie

Ingredients:

- Matcha green tea powder
- Banana, frozen
- Spinach leaves
- Almond milk
- Greek yogurt
- Honey or agave syrup

- Ice cubes

Preparation:

1. In a blender, combine matcha green tea powder, frozen banana, spinach leaves, almond milk, Greek yogurt, honey or agave syrup, and ice cubes.
2. Blend until smooth and creamy.
3. Pour into a glass and enjoy the energizing taste of this matcha green tea smoothie.

Beetroot and Berry Power Juice

Ingredients:

- Beetroot, peeled and chopped
- Mixed berries (strawberries, blueberries, raspberries)
- Carrot, peeled and chopped
- Apple, cored and chopped
- Ginger, peeled
- Water

Preparation:

1. In a juicer, process beetroot, mixed berries, carrot, apple, and ginger.
2. Add water to adjust the consistency if needed.
3. Strain the juice to remove the pulp if desired.
4. Pour into glasses and relish the vibrant and nutritious beetroot and berry power juice.

Chia Seed Lemonade with Honey

Ingredients:

- Chia seeds
- Lemon juice
- Honey
- Water
- Ice cubes
- Lemon slices for garnish

Preparation:

1. In a glass, combine chia seeds, lemon juice, honey, and water.
2. Stir well and let it sit for a few minutes to allow the chia seeds to absorb the liquid.
3. Add ice cubes and stir again.
4. Garnish with lemon slices.
5. Savor this hydrating and textured chia seed lemonade with honey.

Chapter 10: Meal Planning and Grocery Shopping Tips

By strategically organizing your meals and navigating the aisles with purpose, you not only optimize your nutrition but also streamline your culinary journey. Let's explore practical tips and insights that will empower you to make informed choices, save time, and contribute to the overall well-being of your heart.

10.1 Building a Heart-Healthy Grocery List

One of the foundational steps towards fostering a heart-healthy lifestyle is creating a well-curated grocery list. This chapter explores the art of building a grocery list that aligns with your cardiovascular well-being goals, ensuring that your choices in the aisles contribute to a balanced and nutritious diet.

Understanding Heart-Healthy Ingredients:

Begin by familiarizing yourself with heart-healthy ingredients that form the cornerstone of your grocery list. From vibrant fruits and vegetables to lean proteins, whole grains, and heart-friendly fats, having a diverse array of nutrient-rich options lays the groundwork for wholesome meals.

Prioritizing Fresh Produce:

Vegetables and fruits are nutritional powerhouses that should dominate your grocery list. Aim for a colorful assortment, including leafy greens, berries, citrus fruits, and cruciferous vegetables. These provide essential vitamins, minerals, and antioxidants that support heart health.

Selecting Lean Proteins:

Incorporate lean protein sources into your list, such as skinless poultry, fish, legumes, and tofu. These options are rich in protein without the excess saturated fats found in some red meats. Consider variety to ensure a broad spectrum of amino acids.

Opting for Whole Grains:

Swap refined grains for whole grains to enhance the nutritional content of your meals. Quinoa, brown rice, oats, and whole wheat products offer fiber, vitamins, and minerals, contributing to heart health and overall well-being.

Embracing Heart-Friendly Fats:

Include heart-friendly fats like avocados, olive oil, and nuts on your list. These fats, high in monounsaturated and polyunsaturated fats, have been associated with positive cardiovascular effects. Be mindful of portions to maintain a balanced diet.

Navigating Dairy and Dairy Alternatives:

Choose low-fat or fat-free dairy products for calcium and additional nutrients. For those opting for dairy alternatives, fortified options like almond or soy milk can be heart-healthy alternatives.

Exploring the Perimeter of the Grocery Store:

When creating your list, focus on the perimeter of the grocery store where fresh produce, lean proteins, and dairy products are typically located. This strategy helps you prioritize whole, unprocessed foods that contribute to heart health.

Considering Portion Control:

Incorporate portion control into your planning by purchasing appropriately-sized quantities. This not only helps prevent food waste but also supports mindful eating, a key component of a heart-healthy lifestyle.

Checking Labels for Added Sugars and Sodium:

When selecting packaged items, scrutinize food labels for added sugars and sodium. Opt for products with minimal processing and those that align with heart-healthy dietary guidelines.

Creating a Weekly Meal Plan:

To optimize your grocery list, consider planning your meals for the week. This helps streamline your shopping experience and ensures that you have all the necessary ingredients for a balanced and heart-conscious diet.

By focusing on building a heart-healthy grocery list, you lay the foundation for making nutritious and mindful choices in your daily meals. Join me in the next section as we delve into effective meal-planning strategies that bring this thoughtful grocery list to life.

10.2 Weekly Meal Planning for Seniors

Meal planning is a powerful tool, especially for seniors aiming to prioritize heart health. In this section, we explore practical strategies for weekly meal planning tailored to the unique nutritional needs and preferences of seniors. By incorporating a variety of nutrient-rich foods and considering factors such as portion control, we can create well-balanced and heart-healthy meal plans for the week.

Understanding Senior Nutritional Needs:

Begin by acknowledging the specific nutritional needs of seniors. As we age, factors such as reduced metabolism, changes in appetite, and potential health conditions necessitate a thoughtful approach to meal planning. Prioritize foods rich in essential nutrients, including fiber, vitamins, and minerals crucial for heart health and overall well-being.

Incorporating Lean Proteins:

Seniors benefit from adequate protein intake to support muscle health and overall vitality. Include lean protein sources such as fish, poultry, beans, and tofu in your weekly meal plan. Consider varying protein options to ensure a broad spectrum of essential amino acids.

Prioritizing Whole Grains:

Opt for whole grains to provide seniors with sustained energy and important nutrients. Include choices like brown rice, quinoa, whole wheat pasta, and oats in meals to enhance the fiber content and promote digestive health.

Emphasizing Colorful Fruits and Vegetables:

Encourage a vibrant and nutrient-rich diet by incorporating a variety of colorful fruits and vegetables. These foods are packed with antioxidants, vitamins, and minerals essential for heart health. Aim for a rainbow of produce to maximize nutritional benefits.

Mindful Portion Control:

Seniors may find that their appetite and energy needs change over time. Practice mindful portion control by adapting serving sizes to individual requirements. This approach supports weight management and ensures that seniors receive the necessary nutrients without overeating.

Adapting to Dietary Restrictions:

Consider any dietary restrictions or health conditions when planning meals for seniors. Tailor the meal plan to accommodate specific needs, such as reduced sodium intake or restrictions on certain food groups. Consult with healthcare professionals if necessary.

Exploring Culinary Variety:

Enhance the enjoyment of meals by incorporating culinary variety. Experiment with different cooking methods, herbs, and spices to add flavor without relying on excessive salt or unhealthy fats. This variety not only makes meals more interesting but also ensures a broader range of nutrients.

Balancing Meals Throughout the Day:

Distribute nutrients evenly throughout the day by planning balanced meals and snacks. This approach helps maintain stable blood sugar levels and provides a sustained source of energy, contributing to overall health and well-being.

Hydration and Beverage Choices:

Include hydration as an integral part of the meal plan. Encourage seniors to drink an adequate amount of water throughout the day and consider incorporating heart-healthy beverages such as herbal teas and infused water.

Creating a Weekly Meal Calendar:

Organize your meal plan with a weekly calendar, noting breakfast, lunch, dinner, and snacks. This visual aid simplifies grocery shopping and ensures that a diverse array of nutrients is incorporated into daily meals.

Collaborative Planning and Social Engagement:

Consider involving seniors in the meal planning process to align choices with personal preferences. Additionally, meals can be a social experience. Engage in shared cooking or dining activities, promoting a sense of community and enjoyment.

By adopting these principles of weekly meal planning for seniors, we aim to create not just nourishing meals but also an enjoyable and heart-healthy culinary experience. Join me in the next section as we explore practical grocery shopping tips to complement your thoughtful meal plans.

10.3 30-Day Heart-Healthy Meal Plan for Seniors

Week 1:

Day 1

Breakfast (Classic Overnight Oats): 300 Calories | 45g Carbs | 10g Protein | 8g Fat

Lunch (Grilled Chicken Salad): 400 Calories | 20g Carbs | 30g Protein | 15g Fat

Dinner (Baked Salmon with Quinoa): 450 Calories | 30g Carbs | 25g Protein | 20g Fat

Dessert (Dark Chocolate-Dipped Strawberries): 100 Calories | 15g Carbs | 1g Protein | 5g Fat

Snack (Roasted Garlic Hummus): 100 Calories | 10g Carbs | 5g Protein | 6g Fat

Beverage (Green Tea Infusion): 0 Calories | 0g Carbs | 0g Protein | 0g Fat

Day 2

Breakfast (Spinach and Feta Egg Muffins): 250 Calories | 8g Carbs | 20g Protein | 15g Fat

Lunch (Quinoa and Black Bean Bowl): 350 Calories | 50g Carbs | 15g Protein | 8g Fat

Dinner (Sweet Potato and Black Bean Quesadilla): 400 Calories | 60g Carbs | 20g Protein | 10g Fat

Dessert (Oatmeal Banana Cookies): 120 Calories | 15g Carbs | 2g Protein | 6g Fat

Snack (Caprese Skewers): 150 Calories | 8g Carbs | 10g Protein | 10g Fat

Beverage (Berry Blast Smoothie): 200 Calories | 30g Carbs | 8g Protein | 5g Fat

Day 3

Breakfast (Greek Yogurt and Berry Popsicles): 120 Calories | 15g Carbs | 3g Protein | 5g Fat

Lunch (Mediterranean Chickpea Wrap): 350 Calories | 40g Carbs | 15g Protein | 15g Fat

Dinner (Vegetarian Buddha Bowl): 380 Calories | 50g Carbs | 20g Protein | 15g Fat

Dessert (Avocado Chocolate Mousse): 180 Calories | 15g Carbs | 3g Protein

| 12g Fat

Snack (Guacamole with Whole Grain Tortilla Chips): 200 Calories | 20g Carbs | 4g Protein | 12g Fat

Beverage (Hibiscus and Ginger Iced Tea): 30 Calories | 8g Carbs | 0g Protein | 0g Fat

Day 4

Breakfast (Almond Flour Blueberry Muffins): 180 Calories | 20g Carbs | 4g Protein | 10g Fat

Lunch (Caprese Avocado Toast): 320 Calories | 25g Carbs | 10g Protein | 20g Fat

Dinner (Salmon and Quinoa Stuffed Bell Peppers): 420 Calories | 40g Carbs | 30g Protein | 18g Fat

Dessert (Coconut and Berry Chia Seed Pudding): 150 Calories | 15g Carbs | 3g Protein | 8g Fat

Snack (Quinoa-Stuffed Mushrooms): 160 Calories | 15g Carbs | 6g Protein | 8g Fat

Beverage (Kale and Pineapple Detox Juice): 100 Calories | 25g Carbs | 2g Protein | 0g Fat

Day 5

Breakfast (Chia Seed and Mango Parfait): 280 Calories | 30g Carbs | 8g Protein | 15g Fat

Lunch (Turkey and Veggie Lettuce Wraps): 300 Calories | 20g Carbs | 25g Protein | 15g Fat

Dinner (Chickpea and Vegetable Stir-Fry): 380 Calories | 50g Carbs | 15g Protein | 15g Fat

Dessert (Dark Chocolate and Almond Clusters): 120 Calories | 10g Carbs | 3g Protein | 8g Fat

Snack (Cheese and Whole Wheat Crackers Platter): 200 Calories | 15g Carbs | 10g Protein | 12g Fat

Beverage (Golden Turmeric Latte): 150 Calories | 20g Carbs | 5g Protein | 6g Fat

Day 6

Breakfast (Whole Wheat Banana Bread): 230 Calories | 35g Carbs | 3g Protein | 10g Fat

Lunch (Pomegranate and Pistachio Yogurt Parfait): 280 Calories | 25g Carbs | 10g Protein | 15g Fat

Dinner (Quinoa and Black Bean Stuffed Peppers): 400 Calories | 50g Carbs | 20g Protein | 15g Fat

Dessert (Mango Sorbet): 120 Calories | 30g Carbs | 1g Protein | 0g Fat

Snack (Roasted Chickpeas): 150 Calories | 20g Carbs | 6g Protein | 5g Fat

Beverage (Cucumber Basil Sparkling Water): 0 Calories | 0g Carbs | 0g Protein | 0g Fat

Day 7

Breakfast (Mixed Berry Yogurt Parfait): 300 Calories | 40g Carbs | 10g Protein | 12g Fat

Lunch (Lentil and Vegetable Curry with Brown Rice): 380 Calories | 60g Carbs | 18g Protein | 8g Fat

Dinner (Baked Sweet Potato Fries): 250 Calories | 40g Carbs | 3g Protein | 8g Fat

Dessert (Pecan and Date Energy Bites): 180 Calories | 20g Carbs | 3g Protein | 10g Fat

Snack (Veggie Spring Rolls with Peanut Dipping Sauce): 200 Calories | 30g Carbs | 5g Protein | 8g Fat

Beverage (Matcha Green Tea Smoothie): 180 Calories | 15g Carbs | 5g Protein | 10g Fat

Week 2:

Day 8

Breakfast (Banana Walnut Pancakes): 320 Calories | 45g Carbs | 10g Protein | 12g Fat

Lunch (Whole Wheat Veggie Pasta Salad): 380 Calories | 60g Carbs | 15g Protein | 10g Fat

Dinner (Chickpea and Spinach Stew over Couscous): 420 Calories | 70g Carbs | 20g Protein | 8g Fat

Dessert (Almond Flour Blueberry Muffins): 180 Calories | 20g Carbs | 4g Protein | 10g Fat

Snack (Cheese and Whole Wheat Crackers Platter): 200 Calories | 15g Carbs | 10g Protein | 12g Fat

Beverage (Golden Turmeric Latte): 150 Calories | 20g Carbs | 5g Protein | 6g Fat

Day 9

Breakfast (Apple Cinnamon Chia Pudding): 280 Calories | 35g Carbs | 8g Protein | 12g Fat

Lunch (Sweet Potato and Black Bean Quesadilla): 400 Calories | 60g Carbs | 20g Protein | 15g Fat

Dinner (Mediterranean Baked Cod with Tomato and Olive Relish): 380 Calories | 20g Carbs | 30g Protein | 18g Fat

Dessert (Coconut and Berry Chia Seed Pudding): 150 Calories | 15g Carbs | 3g Protein | 8g Fat

Snack (Roasted Chickpeas): 150 Calories | 20g Carbs | 6g Protein | 5g Fat

Beverage (Hibiscus and Ginger Iced Tea): 30 Calories | 8g Carbs | 0g Protein | 0g Fat

Day 10

Breakfast (Veggie and Hummus Breakfast Wrap): 300 Calories | 35g Carbs | 10g Protein | 14g Fat

Lunch (Quinoa and Black Bean Bowl): 350 Calories | 50g Carbs | 15g Protein | 8g Fat

Dinner (Teriyaki Tofu Stir-Fry with Broccoli and Brown Rice): 420 Calories | 55g Carbs | 20g Protein | 14g Fat

Dessert (Dark Chocolate-Dipped Strawberries): 100 Calories | 15g Carbs | 1g Protein | 5g Fat

Snack (Caprese Skewers): 150 Calories | 8g Carbs | 10g Protein | 10g Fat

Beverage (Berry Blast Smoothie): 200 Calories | 30g Carbs | 8g Protein | 5g Fat

Day 11

Breakfast (Pomegranate and Pistachio Yogurt Parfait): 280 Calories | 25g Carbs | 10g Protein | 15g Fat

Lunch (Cauliflower Rice Bowl with Teriyaki Tofu): 380 Calories | 50g Carbs | 20g Protein | 12g Fat

Dinner (Zucchini Noodles with Pesto and Cherry Tomatoes): 350 Calories | 25g Carbs | 8g Protein | 20g Fat

Dessert (Oatmeal Banana Cookies): 120 Calories | 15g Carbs | 2g Protein | 6g Fat

Snack (Guacamole with Whole Grain Tortilla Chips): 200 Calories | 20g Carbs | 4g Protein | 12g Fat

Beverage (Kale and Pineapple Detox Juice): 100 Calories | 25g Carbs | 2g Protein | 0g Fat

Day 12

Breakfast (Salmon and Avocado Bagel): 380 Calories | 40g Carbs | 20g Protein | 18g Fat

Lunch (Roasted Vegetable and Hummus Wrap): 320 Calories | 40g Carbs | 10g Protein | 15g Fat

Dinner (Butternut Squash and Kale Risotto): 420 Calories | 70g Carbs | 12g Protein | 10g Fat

Dessert (Avocado Chocolate Mousse): 180 Calories | 15g Carbs | 3g Protein | 12g Fat

Snack (Quinoa-Stuffed Mushrooms): 160 Calories | 15g Carbs | 6g Protein | 8g Fat

Beverage (Matcha Green Tea Smoothie): 180 Calories | 15g Carbs | 5g Protein | 10g Fat

Day 13

Breakfast (Coconut and Mango Chia Seed Smoothie Bowl): 350 Calories | 45g Carbs | 8g Protein | 18g Fat

Lunch (Tuna and White Bean Salad): 320 Calories | 30g Carbs | 25g Protein | 14g Fat

Dinner (Turkey and Vegetable Skewers with Quinoa Pilaf): 400 Calories | 40g Carbs | 30g Protein | 15g Fat

Dessert (Dark Chocolate and Almond Clusters): 120 Calories | 10g Carbs | 3g Protein | 8g Fat

Snack (Cheese and Whole Wheat Crackers Platter): 200 Calories | 15g Carbs | 10g Protein | 12g Fat

Beverage (Golden Turmeric Latte): 150 Calories | 20g Carbs | 5g Protein | 6g Fat

Day 14

Breakfast (Tomato Basil Mozzarella Frittata): 300 Calories | 25g Carbs | 20g Protein | 15g Fat

Lunch (Cucumber and Greek Yogurt Dip): 250 Calories | 15g Carbs | 8g Protein | 18g Fat

Dinner (Eggplant Parmesan with Whole Wheat Spaghetti): 450 Calories |

60g Carbs | 20g Protein | 16g Fat

Dessert (Mango Sorbet): 120 Calories | 30g Carbs | 1g Protein | 0g Fat

Snack (Baked Parmesan Zucchini Chips): 150 Calories | 10g Carbs | 5g Protein | 12g Fat

Beverage (Hibiscus and Ginger Iced Tea): 30 Calories | 8g Carbs | 0g Protein | 0g Fat

Week 3:

Day 15

Breakfast (Almond Butter Banana Toast): 250 Calories | 30g Carbs | 7g Protein | 12g Fat

Lunch (Greek Quinoa Salad with Grilled Shrimp): 400 Calories | 40g Carbs | 25g Protein | 15g Fat

Dinner (Grilled Salmon with Quinoa and Asparagus): 450 Calories | 30g Carbs | 25g Protein | 20g Fat

Dessert (Chia Seed and Mango Parfait): 280 Calories | 30g Carbs | 8g Protein | 15g Fat

Snack (Roasted Chickpeas): 150 Calories | 20g Carbs | 6g Protein | 5g Fat

Beverage (Berry Blast Smoothie with Flaxseed): 200 Calories | 30g Carbs | 8g Protein | 5g Fat

Day 16

Breakfast (Mediterranean Breakfast Bowl): 300 Calories | 25g Carbs | 15g Protein | 16g Fat

Lunch (Caprese Avocado Toast): 320 Calories | 25g Carbs | 10g Protein | 20g Fat

Dinner (Spinach and Feta Stuffed Chicken Breast with Sweet Potato Mash): 400 Calories | 30g Carbs | 35g Protein | 18g Fat

Dessert (Oatmeal Banana Cookies): 120 Calories | 15g Carbs | 2g Protein |

6g Fat

Snack (Caprese Skewers): 150 Calories | 8g Carbs | 10g Protein | 10g Fat

Beverage (Watermelon Mint Refresher): 100 Calories | 25g Carbs | 0g Protein | 0g Fat

Day 17

Breakfast (Quinoa Breakfast Bowl): 350 Calories | 40g Carbs | 15g Protein | 18g Fat

Lunch (Turkey and Veggie Lettuce Wraps): 300 Calories | 20g Carbs | 25g Protein | 15g Fat

Dinner (Chickpea and Spinach Stew over Couscous): 420 Calories | 70g Carbs | 20g Protein | 8g Fat

Dessert (Dark Chocolate-Dipped Strawberries): 100 Calories | 15g Carbs | 1g Protein | 5g Fat

Snack (Guacamole with Whole Grain Tortilla Chips): 200 Calories | 20g Carbs | 4g Protein | 12g Fat

Beverage (Blueberry and Almond Milk Protein Shake): 200 Calories | 15g Carbs | 10g Protein | 12g Fat

Day 18

Breakfast (Banana Walnut Pancakes): 320 Calories | 45g Carbs | 10g Protein | 12g Fat

Lunch (Whole Wheat Veggie Pasta Salad): 380 Calories | 60g Carbs | 15g Protein | 10g Fat

Dinner (Teriyaki Tofu Stir-Fry with Broccoli and Brown Rice): 420 Calories | 55g Carbs | 20g Protein | 14g Fat

Dessert (Almond Flour Blueberry Muffins): 180 Calories | 20g Carbs | 4g Protein | 10g Fat

Snack (Cheese and Whole Wheat Crackers Platter): 200 Calories | 15g Carbs | 10g Protein | 12g Fat

Beverage (Golden Turmeric Latte): 150 Calories | 20g Carbs | 5g Protein |

6g Fat

Day 19

Breakfast (Apple Cinnamon Chia Pudding): 280 Calories | 35g Carbs | 8g Protein | 12g Fat

Lunch (Sweet Potato and Black Bean Quesadilla): 400 Calories | 60g Carbs | 20g Protein | 15g Fat

Dinner (Mediterranean Baked Cod with Tomato and Olive Relish): 380 Calories | 20g Carbs | 30g Protein | 18g Fat

Dessert (Coconut and Berry Chia Seed Pudding): 150 Calories | 15g Carbs | 3g Protein | 8g Fat

Snack (Roasted Chickpeas): 150 Calories | 20g Carbs | 6g Protein | 5g Fat

Beverage (Hibiscus and Ginger Iced Tea): 30 Calories | 8g Carbs | 0g Protein | 0g Fat

Day 20

Breakfast (Veggie and Hummus Breakfast Wrap): 300 Calories | 35g Carbs | 10g Protein | 14g Fat

Lunch (Quinoa and Black Bean Bowl): 350 Calories | 50g Carbs | 15g Protein | 8g Fat

Dinner (Roasted Vegetable and Hummus Wrap): 320 Calories | 40g Carbs | 10g Protein | 15g Fat

Dessert (Dark Chocolate-Dipped Strawberries): 100 Calories | 15g Carbs | 1g Protein | 5g Fat

Snack (Caprese Skewers): 150 Calories | 8g Carbs | 10g Protein | 10g Fat

Beverage (Berry Blast Smoothie): 200 Calories | 30g Carbs | 8g Protein | 5g Fat

Day 21:

Breakfast (Mediterranean Breakfast Bowl): 300 Calories | 25g Carbs | 15g

Protein | 16g Fat

Lunch (Caprese Avocado Toast): 320 Calories | 25g Carbs | 10g Protein | 20g Fat

Dinner (Spinach and Feta Stuffed Chicken Breast with Sweet Potato Mash): 400 Calories | 30g Carbs | 35g Protein | 18g Fat

Dessert (Oatmeal Banana Cookies): 120 Calories | 15g Carbs | 2g Protein | 6g Fat

Snack (Caprese Skewers): 150 Calories | 8g Carbs | 10g Protein | 10g Fat

Beverage (Watermelon Mint Refresher): 100 Calories | 25g Carbs | 0g Protein | 0g Fat

Week 4:

Day 22:

Breakfast (Quinoa Breakfast Bowl): 350 Calories | 40g Carbs | 15g Protein | 18g Fat

Lunch (Turkey and Veggie Lettuce Wraps): 300 Calories | 20g Carbs | 25g Protein | 15g Fat

Dinner (Chickpea and Spinach Stew over Couscous): 420 Calories | 70g Carbs | 20g Protein | 8g Fat

Dessert (Dark Chocolate-Dipped Strawberries): 100 Calories | 15g Carbs | 1g Protein | 5g Fat

Snack (Guacamole with Whole Grain Tortilla Chips): 200 Calories | 20g Carbs | 4g Protein | 12g Fat

Beverage (Blueberry and Almond Milk Protein Shake): 200 Calories | 15g Carbs | 10g Protein | 12g Fat

Day 23:

Breakfast (Banana Walnut Pancakes): 320 Calories | 45g Carbs | 10g Protein |

12g Fat

Lunch (Whole Wheat Veggie Pasta Salad): 380 Calories | 60g Carbs | 15g Protein | 10g Fat

Dinner (Teriyaki Tofu Stir-Fry with Broccoli and Brown Rice): 420 Calories | 55g Carbs | 20g Protein | 14g Fat

Dessert (Almond Flour Blueberry Muffins): 180 Calories | 20g Carbs | 4g Protein | 10g Fat

Snack (Cheese and Whole Wheat Crackers Platter): 200 Calories | 15g Carbs | 10g Protein | 12g Fat

Beverage (Golden Turmeric Latte): 150 Calories | 20g Carbs | 5g Protein | 6g Fat

Day 24:

Breakfast (Apple Cinnamon Chia Pudding): 280 Calories | 35g Carbs | 8g Protein | 12g Fat

Lunch (Sweet Potato and Black Bean Quesadilla): 400 Calories | 60g Carbs | 20g Protein | 15g Fat

Dinner (Mediterranean Baked Cod with Tomato and Olive Relish): 380 Calories | 20g Carbs | 30g Protein | 18g Fat

Dessert (Coconut and Berry Chia Seed Pudding): 150 Calories | 15g Carbs | 3g Protein | 8g Fat

Snack (Roasted Chickpeas): 150 Calories | 20g Carbs | 6g Protein | 5g Fat

Beverage (Hibiscus and Ginger Iced Tea): 30 Calories | 8g Carbs | 0g Protein | 0g Fat

Day 25:

Breakfast (Veggie and Hummus Breakfast Wrap): 300 Calories | 35g Carbs | 10g Protein | 14g Fat

Lunch (Quinoa and Black Bean Bowl): 350 Calories | 50g Carbs | 15g Protein | 8g Fat

Dinner (Roasted Vegetable and Hummus Wrap): 320 Calories | 40g Carbs |

10g Protein | 15g Fat

Dessert (Dark Chocolate-Dipped Strawberries): 100 Calories | 15g Carbs | 1g Protein | 5g Fat

Snack (Caprese Skewers): 150 Calories | 8g Carbs | 10g Protein | 10g Fat

Beverage (Berry Blast Smoothie): 200 Calories | 30g Carbs | 8g Protein | 5g Fat

Day 26:

Breakfast (Coconut and Mango Chia Seed Smoothie Bowl): 350 Calories | 45g Carbs | 8g Protein | 18g Fat

Lunch (Tuna and White Bean Salad): 320 Calories | 30g Carbs | 25g Protein | 14g Fat

Dinner (Turkey and Vegetable Skewers with Quinoa Pilaf): 400 Calories | 40g Carbs | 30g Protein | 15g Fat

Dessert (Dark Chocolate and Almond Clusters): 120 Calories | 10g Carbs | 3g Protein | 8g Fat

Snack (Cheese and Whole Wheat Crackers Platter): 200 Calories | 15g Carbs | 10g Protein | 12g Fat

Beverage (Golden Turmeric Latte): 150 Calories | 20g Carbs | 5g Protein | 6g Fat

Day 27:

Breakfast (Tomato Basil Mozzarella Frittata): 300 Calories | 25g Carbs | 20g Protein | 15g Fat

Lunch (Cucumber and Greek Yogurt Dip): 250 Calories | 15g Carbs | 8g Protein | 18g Fat

Dinner (Eggplant Parmesan with Whole Wheat Spaghetti): 450 Calories | 60g Carbs | 20g Protein | 16g Fat

Dessert (Mango Sorbet): 120 Calories | 30g Carbs | 1g Protein | 0g Fat

Snack (Baked Parmesan Zucchini Chips): 150 Calories | 10g Carbs | 5g Protein | 12g Fat

Beverage (Hibiscus and Ginger Iced Tea): 30 Calories | 8g Carbs | 0g Protein | 0g Fat

Day 28:

Breakfast (Classic Overnight Oats): 300 Calories | 40g Carbs | 10g Protein | 12g Fat

Lunch (Grilled Chicken Salad with Mixed Greens): 350 Calories | 25g Carbs | 30g Protein | 15g Fat

Dinner (Baked Lemon Herb Chicken with Roasted Vegetables): 400 Calories | 35g Carbs | 30g Protein | 18g Fat

Dessert (Chia Seed and Mango Parfait): 280 Calories | 30g Carbs | 8g Protein | 15g Fat

Snack (Roasted Garlic Hummus with Veggie Sticks): 150 Calories | 15g Carbs | 6g Protein | 8g Fat

Beverage (Green Tea Infusion with Citrus Twist): 0 Calories | 0g Carbs | 0g Protein | 0g Fat

Day 29:

Breakfast (Spinach and Feta Egg Muffins): 250 Calories | 15g Carbs | 15g Protein | 15g Fat

Lunch (Quinoa and Black Bean Bowl): 350 Calories | 50g Carbs | 15g Protein | 8g Fat

Dinner (Grilled Salmon with Quinoa and Asparagus): 450 Calories | 30g Carbs | 25g Protein | 20g Fat

Dessert (Almond Flour Blueberry Muffins): 180 Calories | 20g Carbs | 4g Protein | 10g Fat

Snack (Caprese Skewers): 150 Calories | 8g Carbs | 10g Protein | 10g Fat

Beverage (Golden Turmeric Latte): 150 Calories | 20g Carbs | 5g Protein | 6g Fat

Day 30:

Breakfast (Smashed Avocado on Whole-Grain Toast with Cherry Tomatoes): 280 Calories | 30g Carbs | 6g Protein | 18g Fat

Lunch (Caprese Avocado Toast): 320 Calories | 25g Carbs | 10g Protein | 20g Fat

Dinner (Spinach and Feta Stuffed Chicken Breast with Sweet Potato Mash): 400 Calories | 30g Carbs | 35g Protein | 18g Fat

Dessert (Oatmeal Banana Cookies): 120 Calories | 15g Carbs | 2g Protein | 6g Fat

Snack (Caprese Skewers): 150 Calories | 8g Carbs | 10g Protein | 10g Fat

Beverage (Watermelon Mint Refresher): 100 Calories | 25g Carbs | 0g Protein | 0g Fat

Chapter 11: Maintaining a Heart-Healthy Lifestyle

Living a heart-healthy lifestyle is not just about the food you eat but extends to various aspects of your daily routine. In this chapter, we'll explore key practices and habits that contribute to cardiovascular well-being, ensuring that the principles outlined in this cookbook become an integral part of your life.

11.1 Incorporating Physical Activity

Physical activity is a fundamental aspect of maintaining a healthy heart. In this section, we'll explore practical ways to incorporate regular exercise into your daily life, promoting cardiovascular fitness and overall well-being.

1. Choose Activities You Enjoy:

Opt for activities that bring you joy and excitement. Whether it's walking, dancing, swimming, or cycling, selecting exercises you love increases the likelihood that you'll stick with them.

2. Start Slow and Gradual:

If you're new to exercise or returning after a hiatus, begin with low-intensity activities. Gradually increase the duration and intensity over time to avoid overexertion and injuries.

3. Set Realistic Goals:

Establish achievable fitness goals. Whether it's walking a certain number of steps per day or completing a specific workout routine, realistic goals help you stay motivated and build a sustainable exercise routine.

4. Make it a Social Activity:

Engage in physical activities with friends or family. This not only adds a social element to your exercise routine but can also make it more enjoyable and provide mutual motivation.

5. Integrate Exercise into Daily Life:

Look for opportunities to move throughout the day. Take the stairs instead of the elevator, walk or bike for short errands, or engage in quick stretching exercises during breaks.

6. Schedule Regular Workouts:

Treat your exercise sessions as important appointments. Schedule them into your calendar to create a routine, making it more likely that you'll prioritize and commit to regular physical activity.

7. Mix Up Your Routine:

Keep your exercise routine interesting by incorporating a variety of activities. This not only prevents boredom but also ensures that different muscle groups are engaged, promoting overall fitness.

8. Consider Strength Training:

Include strength training exercises at least two days a week. This could involve using weights, resistance bands, or bodyweight exercises to enhance muscle strength and support joint health.

9. Listen to Your Body:

Pay attention to how your body responds to exercise. If you experience pain or discomfort, adjust your routine accordingly. It's essential to find a balance between challenging yourself and avoiding injury.

10. Stay Consistent:

Consistency is key to reaping the benefits of physical activity. Aim for at least 150 minutes of moderate-intensity aerobic activity per week, along with muscle-strengthening activities on two or more days.

Incorporating physical activity into your lifestyle doesn't have to be daunting. By making it enjoyable, gradual, and tailored to your preferences, you can cultivate a sustainable exercise routine that contributes to a healthier heart and a more vibrant life.

11.2 Stress Management and Its Impact on Heart Health

In the fast-paced world we live in, managing stress is crucial for maintaining a healthy heart. Chronic stress has been linked to various cardiovascular issues, making stress management an integral component of a heart-healthy lifestyle. In this section, we'll explore the impact of stress on heart health and effective strategies to manage and mitigate its effects.

Understanding the Impact:

Chronic stress triggers the body's "fight or flight" response, releasing stress hormones such as cortisol and adrenaline. While this response is essential in acute situations, prolonged exposure to stress can contribute to:

Elevated Blood Pressure: Chronic stress can lead to sustained high blood pressure, increasing the risk of heart disease and stroke.

Inflammation: Stress may contribute to inflammation in the body, a factor associated with heart disease.

Unhealthy Behaviors: Individuals under stress may resort to unhealthy coping mechanisms such as smoking, overeating, or excessive alcohol consumption, further impacting heart health.

Effective Stress Management Strategies:

Mindfulness Meditation: Practice mindfulness meditation to bring awareness to the present moment. This technique has been shown to reduce stress and improve overall well-being.

Deep Breathing Exercises: Incorporate deep breathing exercises into your daily routine. Deep, slow breaths can trigger the body's relaxation response, reducing stress levels.

Regular Physical Activity: Engage in regular exercise, as it not only benefits physical health but also acts as a powerful stress reducer by promoting the release of endorphins.

Healthy Lifestyle Choices: Prioritize a balanced and nutritious diet. Avoid excessive caffeine and sugar intake, as these can contribute to stress and energy fluctuations.

Adequate Sleep: Ensure you get sufficient, quality sleep. Sleep plays a crucial role in stress recovery and overall cardiovascular health.

Social Connections: Foster positive relationships with friends and family. Social support is a valuable resource in times of stress.

Time Management: Organize your schedule and prioritize tasks. Effective time management can reduce feelings of being overwhelmed.

Hobbies and Relaxation Techniques: Engage in activities you enjoy, whether it's reading, gardening, or listening to music. Finding time for hobbies and relaxation is essential for stress relief.

Seeking Professional Support: If stress becomes overwhelming, consider seeking support from a mental health professional. They can provide coping strategies and support tailored to your individual needs.

In Conclusion:

Recognizing the impact of stress on heart health and implementing effective stress management strategies is a proactive step toward maintaining a healthy cardiovascular system. By integrating these practices into your routine, you not only enhance your heart health but also contribute to overall well-being and resilience in the face of life's challenges.

11.3 Regular Health Checkups for Seniors

Regular health checkups are a crucial component of proactive healthcare, especially for seniors. These routine assessments play a pivotal role in early detection, prevention, and management of potential health issues. In this section, we'll explore the importance of regular health checkups for seniors and the key screenings and examinations that contribute to maintaining overall well-being.

Understanding the Importance:

• Early Detection of Health Issues:

Regular checkups allow healthcare professionals to identify potential health issues in their early stages. Early detection often leads to more effective treatment and better health outcomes.

• Preventive Care:

Health checkups provide an opportunity for preventive care measures, such as vaccinations, screenings, and lifestyle recommendations, to help seniors maintain optimal health.

• Management of Chronic Conditions:

For seniors with existing chronic conditions, regular checkups enable healthcare providers to monitor and manage these conditions effectively, preventing complications.

• Medication Management:

Regular checkups allow healthcare professionals to review and adjust medications as needed. This ensures that seniors are on the most effective and appropriate treatment plans.

• Health Risk Assessments:

Comprehensive health checkups often include assessments of lifestyle factors, family history, and other determinants that contribute to a personalized understanding of health risks.

Key Components of Regular Health Checkups for Seniors:

- Blood Pressure Monitoring:

Regular blood pressure checks are essential for detecting and managing hypertension, a common risk factor for heart disease and stroke.

- Cholesterol Levels:

Monitoring cholesterol levels helps assess cardiovascular health and reduce the risk of heart disease.

- Blood Glucose Testing:

Seniors, especially those at risk for diabetes, should undergo regular blood glucose testing to monitor and manage blood sugar levels.

- Cancer Screenings:

Screening for cancers such as breast, colorectal, prostate, and cervical cancers helps in early detection and improved treatment outcomes.

- Bone Density Scan:

For seniors at risk of osteoporosis, bone density scans assess bone health and fracture risk.

- Vision and Hearing Tests:

Regular vision and hearing tests are crucial for maintaining sensory health and addressing issues such as age-related macular degeneration and hearing loss.

- Immunizations:

Stay up-to-date with recommended vaccinations to protect against diseases and infections, including influenza and pneumonia.

- Mental Health Assessment:

Regular mental health checkups help identify and manage conditions such as depression or anxiety, which can impact overall well-being.

- Skin Checks:

Regular examination of the skin aids in the early detection of skin cancers and other dermatological issues.

- Adhering to a Regular Checkup Schedule:

Seniors should work closely with their healthcare providers to establish a regular checkup schedule tailored to their individual health needs. Open communication and active involvement in healthcare decisions contribute to a comprehensive approach to senior well-being.

In conclusion, regular health checkups are a proactive and essential aspect of senior healthcare, fostering early detection, prevention, and effective management of health issues. Prioritizing these checkups empowers seniors to take charge of their health and enjoy a vibrant and fulfilling life.

Chapter 12: Conclusion

In the final chapter of the "Heart Healthy Cookbook for Seniors 2024," we wrap up our culinary journey with gratitude for the opportunity to guide you toward a heart-healthy and fulfilling lifestyle. As we conclude this cookbook, let's reflect on the key takeaways, express appreciation for the journey we've shared, and reinforce the principles that underpin a heart-healthy approach for seniors.

12.1 Celebrating a Heart-Healthy Lifestyle

As we conclude our exploration of heart-healthy living in this chapter, it's time to celebrate the journey you've embarked upon toward a healthier and more vibrant lifestyle. The commitment to heart health is not merely a duty but a celebration of self-care and well-being. In this section, we reflect on the achievements made, acknowledge the positive changes, and embrace the joy that comes with embracing a heart-healthy lifestyle.

Reflecting on Achievements:

Culinary Exploration: By engaging with the diverse and delicious recipes presented in this cookbook, you've embarked on a culinary adventure that combines nutrition with flavor. Each meal prepared and enjoyed is a celebration of your commitment to heart-healthy eating.

Lifestyle Integration: Incorporating physical activity, stress management, and regular health checkups into your routine reflects a holistic approach to heart health. Celebrate the steps you've taken to create a well-rounded and sustainable lifestyle that supports your cardiovascular well-being.

Knowledge Empowerment: Understanding the principles of heart-healthy living empowers you to make informed choices. Celebrate the knowledge gained and the confidence it brings in navigating your health journey.

Acknowledging Positive Changes:

Nourishing Choices: The shift towards incorporating heart-healthy ingredients and cooking techniques into your meals is a positive change that directly impacts your cardiovascular health. Celebrate the nourishing choices you've made for your heart.

Active Living: Whether it's a daily walk, yoga session, or other forms of physical activity, acknowledge the positive change in embracing an active lifestyle. Celebrate the joy of movement and its positive impact on your heart and overall well-being.

Stress Resilience: As you adopt stress management techniques, celebrate your growing resilience. The ability to navigate stress positively is a valuable skill that contributes to heart health and overall mental well-being.

Embracing Joy in the Journey:

Culinary Pleasures: Celebrate the pleasure of savoring delicious and heart-healthy meals. Take joy in the flavors, textures, and nourishment each dish brings to your table.

Active Pursuits: Find joy in the various physical activities you engage in. Whether it's a dance class, a nature hike, or a simple stroll, let the joy of movement be a source of motivation.

Mindful Moments: Embrace moments of mindfulness and relaxation. Celebrate the serenity found in practices such as meditation or deep breathing, nurturing both your mind and heart.

As you celebrate a heart-healthy lifestyle, remember that each positive choice, no matter how small, contributes to a healthier and more fulfilling life. The journey is ongoing, and every step is a cause for celebration. Here's to your heart health, well-being, and the joyous celebration of a life well-lived.

12.2 Final Note

As we conclude this heart-healthy journey together, let this final note be a reminder of the profound impact you can have on your well-being. Your commitment to heart health is a testament to the resilience and care you extend to yourself.

Take a moment to reflect on the steps you've taken, the recipes you've explored, and the mindful choices you've made. Your dedication to a heart-healthy lifestyle is an investment in a future filled with vitality and fulfillment.

We express our heartfelt gratitude for allowing us to be part of your journey. The pursuit of heart health is a shared mission, and your engagement with this cookbook signifies a commitment to a life of well-being.

As you move forward, carry the knowledge gained within these pages as a beacon guiding your choices. Your heart is at the center of your health, and each decision you make is an opportunity to nurture and protect it.

Embrace the joy found in nourishing meals, the vitality gained through movement, and the peace cultivated in moments of reflection. Your heart-healthy lifestyle is not a destination but a continuous journey, and we encourage you to approach it with curiosity, enthusiasm, and a sense of celebration.

Continue to explore, experiment, and find joy in the pursuit of a heart-healthy life. Seek inspiration in new recipes, enjoy the benefits of an active lifestyle, and savor the moments of tranquility that contribute to your overall well-being.

Remember, you are the author of your health story, and every positive choice is a page turned towards a healthier, more vibrant future.

May your heart be filled with gratitude for the journey, hope for the future, and the joy that comes from prioritizing your health. Here's to a heart-full life—a life that beats with energy, nourishment, and the fulfillment that comes from embracing a heart-healthy lifestyle.

Thank you for sharing this journey with us, and may your heart continue to beat in rhythm with the melody of well-being.